LEAH KAMINSKY

Writer, M.D.

Leah Kaminsky is an award-winning writer and a practicing family physician. She is the author of four books, including *Stitching Things Together,* a collection of poetry. She has studied writing at the Iowa Writers' Workshop, New York University, and Vermont College of Fine Arts, and is currently at work on her first novel. She lives in Melbourne, Australia.

Writer, M.D.

Writer, M.D.

The Best Contemporary Fiction and Nonfiction by Doctors

EDITED BY LEAH KAMINSKY

VINTAGE BOOKS

A DIVISION OF RANDOM HOUSE, INC.

NEW YORK

A VINTAGE BOOKS ORIGINAL, JANUARY 2012

Copyright © 2012 by Leah Kaminsky

All rights reserved. Published in the United States by Vintage Books,
a division of Random House, Inc., New York,
and in Canada by Random House of Canada Limited, Toronto.
Originally published, in different form,
in Australia as *The Pen and the Stethoscope*
by Scribe Publications Pty Ltd., Melbourne.

Vintage and colophon are registered trademarks of Random House, Inc.

Owing to limitations of space, permission to reprint previously published
material may be found on pages 253–254.

The Cataloging-in-Publication Data for *Writer, M.D.*
is available at the Library of Congress.

ISBN: 978-0-307-94686-7

Book design by R. Bull

www.vintagebooks.com

Printed in the United States of America
10 9 8 7 6 5 4 3 2 1

For Yohanan, Alon, Ella, and Maia Loeffler

Contents

Medicine is my lawful wife and literature my mistress; when I get tired of one, I spend the night with the other.

—*Anton Chekhov*

Foreword

A physician works at the border between science and the soul. Schooled in physiology and pharmacology, the molecular workings of genes and proteins, the biochemistry of health and disease, a doctor brings to care a diverse body of expert knowledge. That knowledge is rapidly expanding with the use of sophisticated technologies such as genomics that map mutations in our DNA, and MRI scans that reveal millimeter abnormalities in our inner organs. This wealth of information has changed the nature of diagnosis and treatment, bringing many maladies under the bright light of science, illuminating their genesis, and providing a rational basis for their remedy.

But what has not changed over the millennia is the human soul. The role of the physician as healer has not been fundamentally altered by his burgeoning knowledge. Greater knowledge does not necessarily translate into greater wisdom. Wisdom requires melding information with judgment and values. The wise doctor probes not only the organs of his patient but also his feelings and emotions, his fears and his hopes, his regrets and his goals. And to accomplish that most important task of applying wisdom, the physician also needs to take his own emotional temperature, to realize how his own beliefs and biases may be brought to bear in his efforts to secure a better future for his patient.

This remarkable collection melds science and the soul, logic with feeling, knowledge with wisdom. The voices that the reader hears are among the most prominent in the constellation of physician-writers. What makes these writers so compelling is not only the fluidity of their prose and the intensity of their focus, not only their literary and narrative skills, but also their remarkable degree of self-awareness. A physician is trained in medical school and residency to hide his feelings and filter his thoughts. This training is required in order to effectively deliver care in an environment that is often chaotic and unnerving. The doctor needs to present himself to the patient as a safe harbor of stability in the midst of the tempest of illness. But when that doctor has moved from the clinic to the page, the mask drops, and we see the turmoil and tribulations in his heart and mind. The humanity of both patient and physician is what makes the stories that follow so rich and so fulfilling.

Jerome Groopman

Introduction

When I first became a medical student, many years ago, I developed a condition I call Tunnel Vision of the Soul. It is a crippling ailment in which you see only things that are straight in front of you. You focus on the sickness and don't see the sick person. Your peripheral vision is blurred, so that you don't notice your surroundings, with all their inherent colors, nuances, and possibilities, unless you deliberately turn your head to look. The onset can be insidious, the symptoms barely perceptible at first.

As I was spending lunchtimes in the anatomy museum, surrounded by dissections under glass, it never occurred to me that what lay exposed was the pelvis of someone's mother, or the foot of somebody's brother. I munched on chicken sandwiches, busily memorizing mnemonics: Swiftly Lower Tilley's Pants To Try Coitus There, for the bones of the wrist; Grandpa Shagging Grandma's Love Child, for the top layers of the skin.

After six years as a medical student, practicing rectal examinations on old men who had become paralyzed following a stroke, performing bone marrow biopsies on dying little old ladies, and shoving needles into the spines of crying babies, I emerged almost totally desensitized to human pain and suffering. My fortnightly salary checks were based on the fact that other people fell ill, or died.

And as a cocky young intern, proudly wearing my long white coat while strolling through the wards of a large teaching hospital, I felt impermeable.

The cure for my tunnel vision came gradually. I started reading literature, which coaxed me to return to writing—something I hadn't done since high school. With my trembling pen, I began to heal my own wounds and try to make some sort of sense of what I had experienced as a young doctor and as a human being.

Since that time, my medicine has always fed and informed my writing. More important, my writing has hopefully made me a better doctor. Becoming a writer has opened my eyes, so that I am able to see my patients as human beings, each one with his or her very own story to tell. And nowadays, I hope that I am able to listen to their hearts—with both my stethoscope and my pen poised.

Writer, M.D. is a collection of stories—fiction and non-fiction—that aims to look behind the doctor's mask. What goes on inside the mind of the human being who deals with enormous existential issues and traumatic situations on a daily basis? It is through writing that many doctors have plumbed the depths and richness of their experience and, in turn, used this to explore their patients' inner lives.

These stories canvass emotional experiences acutely felt by doctors—an awareness of our mortality, of how humanity interplays with medicine, of the weight of responsibility carried by the profession. The fiction pieces, in particular, often use the point of view of the patient to examine a range of issues, including grief, trauma, illness, and aging.

The public is hungry to see behind the veneer of the medical professional, as evidenced by the burgeoning number of TV shows such as *ER* and *Grey's Anatomy*. This book delves beyond sensationalism, taking a critical look at doctors' close observations of, and reflections upon, their working lives.

Physician-writers have a long tradition. Apollo managed to have a dual career as the Greek god of both poetry and medicine. Copernicus, Maimonides, Bulgakov, and Chekhov were all physicians who purloined their patients' narratives. In this anthology, I hope the reader will be afforded a glimpse of the world through the eyes of some of our best contemporary doctor-writers. Every patient has a story to tell, if only you take the time to listen.

Leah Kaminsky

nonfiction

Bedside Manners

ABRAHAM VERGHESE

When it was time to hang pictures in our new house in San Antonio, my wife asked me to buy a stud finder. As a husband, I demurred; as an internist, I flat-out refused. We internists make it our business to divine the stutters and stumbles of lungs, hearts, brains, adrenals, guts, gonads—hence the term "internal medicine." Once upon a time, doctors examined patients not with CAT scans or MRIs but with their senses. "Surely," I said, "skills that can find pus behind the chest wall can find a stud behind drywall."

Under her skeptical eye, I dragged my fingertips along the wallpaper. I flattened my palm and tapped on the back of my left middle finger using the tip of my right middle finger. My hands drummed over the pressed gypsum, sounding it, discovering the spots where the resonance became muffled, abbreviated—*thud* rather than *thoom*. In the medical world, this is known as percussion, a technique that physicians have employed for centuries to sound the body's depths. Using it, I had found the upright wooden timbers that even in the best circles of society are called studs. My brother-in-law, who fought in Korea, who wears ten-gallon hats, and who is fond of me but feels that most medical professionals are in it for the luxury cars, golf, exotic vacations, and early retirement, was impressed. As we hammered the nails in and hung the pictures, he said, "I didn't think a doctor could do that anymore."

My wife thinks of me as a Luddite. She believes that if a gadget has found its way onto a catalog page, and if its price is many multiples of a bar of soap, it must be useful. But that evening the pendulum swung in my favor. It was one of those man-puts-machines-to-pasture moments where the sheeplike drift of consumer society toward another "must have" is momentarily halted. Please, I beg you, say no to pet dishes on legs that enable Fido to drink in an "anatomically correct" fashion, say no to battery-operated fridge air purifiers, and say no to stud finders. I fell asleep that night thinking about an instructional pamphlet that I would put in every homeowner's Welcome Wagon basket, alongside the coupons, refrigerator magnets, and recipes for orange-peel-flavored scones: "Find the Hidden Stud in Your New Texas Home."

The sad thing is that a homeowner armed with such a pamphlet and with one other critical ingredient—faith—can soon become more skilled at percussion than the average physician. It is fast becoming a lost art. In the past twenty-five years, I have taught hundreds of medical students the four classic steps in the physical examination: inspect, palpate, percuss, and auscultate. Their eyes sparkle. This is the way they imagined themselves: semioticians at the bedside, reading the signs to find the varmint in the patient's body. Alas, a shock awaits the students when they finally arrive on the wards in the third year of medical school, their pockets laden with reflex hammers, tuning forks, ophthalmoscopes, otoscopes, penlights, and stethoscopes, only to discover that the ebb and flow of the modern hospital centers on MRIs, CAT scans, echocardiograms, angiograms, and myriad lab tests. Often, interns

and residents have so little faith in bedside diagnostic skills
that, as one student told me, "a man with a missing finger
must get an X-ray before anyone will believe he has only
four." As for neat pocket tools, only a few diehards still
carry them. The stethoscope alone peeks out of the doctor's pocket as a hollow symbol of the profession. (I prefer
seeing it in the pocket to seeing it draped over the neck
like the beads and gris-gris of Wodaabe tribesmen of the
Sahara, a vulgar display meant to signal that the wearer is
a sound marriage prospect and has, if not cows and land,
then the prospect of luxury cars, golf, exotic vacations,
and early retirement.)

When I travel as a visiting professor to teaching hospitals, I have the distinct feeling that the patient in America is
becoming invisible. She is unseen and unheard. She is "presented" to me by the intern and resident team in a conference room far away from where she lies. Her illness has
been translated into binary signals stored in the computer.
When I ask a question about her, the intern's head instinctively turns to the computer screen, like a pitcher checking
first base. I gently insist we go to the bedside, but that is
often a place where the team is no longer at ease. I realize
what has happened: the patient in the bed is merely an icon
for the real patient, who exists in the computer. How strange
this is! When one knows how to look, the patient's body is
an illuminated manuscript. Indeed, in an elderly patient
with a double-digit "problem list" that scrolls off the screen,
only at the bedside does one understand which problem is
most important. As my brother-in-law would put it, "You
have to kick the tires."

I am no economist, but even a landlubber on a sinking ship
is entitled to make observations about the rent in the hull that
is about to alter his fate: the present crisis in American health

care is only secondarily a fiscal one; the real crisis is that the "art" of bedside diagnosis at which a previous generation excelled has died with the next. Personal-injury lawyers allow us the wonderful excuse that we order batteries of tests because we are practicing "defensive" medicine. The truth is that, even without the threat of malpractice, we would still need just as many CAT scans and echocardiograms as we do now. We know no other way. Take away our stud finders and we can't hang a picture. We are like owners of playerless pianos asked to entertain during a blackout: our fingers and ears may be intact, but we can no longer play or percuss.

It was an innkeeper's son, Josef Leopold Auenbrugger, who discovered percussion. I have dreamed this scene so often that I am convinced it must have happened. Imagine Vienna in the eighteenth century:

The inn is bustling. Young Josef and his father carry empty wine jugs down to the cellar. Auenbrugger père hums as he descends, the sound enlarging in the cool cavern, where three large casks of wine sit like three portly giants. Since the casks are not transparent, the question is always how much wine remains inside each one.

Auenbrugger père raps with his knuckles on the side of each cask. At the top he generates a hollow sound, a profundo, like a bass drum. As his knuckles come down the side, there is a point where the sound changes. The sustained echo—the thoom—*is stifled, and the new sound is dull and flat, as if the old sound were decapitated. Young Josef, just like his father, "sees" through the cask, where the reflective, liquid surface ripples at his touch.*

In Auenbrugger's time, physicians focused largely on symptoms, and had no great need to touch the patient (which some would argue is where we are now). Knowing what ailed you made little difference because, as far as treatment went, you could only be cupped, purged, scari-fied, or bled. Bleeding was to that era what antibiotics are to ours: abundant and overused. At the barber-surgeon's establishment, you held on to a pole as he sliced you and collected your blood in a basin. While there, you could also get a tooth pulled, an abscess drained, and finish up with a shave and a haircut. The barber-surgeon was nothing if not versatile. At the end of the day, the barbers washed long strips of bandage and hung them outside to dry. Medical students are often surprised when I tell them that the familiar red-and-white barber's pole has its origins in bloodletting, with the stripes represent-ing the bloody bandages and the ball on the top of the pole representing the basin. If you had a chance to live, these treatments might nevertheless do you in; if you were destined to die, they mercifully hastened the end.

When Auenbrugger became a physician, he started thumping and tapping on his patients, and painstakingly cataloging the sounds of health and disease they produced. The book he wrote about this practice, *Inventum novum*, published in 1761, had the impact on medicine that X-rays would have 150 years later. For the first time, a doctor could "see" beneath the intact skin into the innards of the body. Percussion allowed (and still allows) a physician to get evi-dence of a dilated heart, an enlarged liver, fluid around the lung, fluid in the belly, a perforated stomach ulcer, and many other conditions. I think of present-day ultrasound as the child of percussion, the ultrasound transducer generat-ing a sound wave that bounces off the tissues and comes back to a sensor.

Like any new method, percussion had its overenthusias-tic practitioners. The famous Pierre Piorry percussed while sitting on a high stool next to the patient's bed, and then used colored crayons to outline the organs. Known as the "medical Paganini," Piorry claimed each organ had its own note and the body held a musical scale. An apocryphal story has Piorry going to see the king and, on being told that the king was out, proceeding to percuss the chamber door and declare that the king was in.

I attended medical school on two continents. My first clinical professor in Addis Ababa, Ethiopia, was a spiritual descendant of Auenbrugger's named Charles Leithead. He taught us how to place our fingers on the wrists of patients with rheumatic heart-valve disease and recognize the slapping, "water hammer" pulse of a leaky aortic valve or the "plateau pulse" (pulsus parvus et tardus) of a narrowed aortic valve. He marched us to the heart, taking the blood pressure along the way, studying the sinuous waveforms of the neck veins, which mirrored the happenings in the heart's upper chamber. He carefully inspected the patient's chest and felt for the thrust of the heart between the fifth and sixth ribs on the left, though in an enlarged heart, the impulse could wander down and out to the armpit. At this point in an exam, he had us pause and try to put the clues together. His teaching was: "Before you pull out your stethoscope, you should know what you are going to hear." It was heady, marvelous stuff. When I finally heard the soft, rumbling, low-pitched, mid-diastolic murmur of mitral valve narrowing that is caught only with the bell of the stethoscope lightly applied, I was ecstatic. I heard it because I knew it would be there.

Displaced from Africa by civil strife, I went to Madras, in South India, to finish my studies. My teacher was the legendary K. V. Thiruvengadam, known to all as KVT. KVT is the Ravi Shankar of percussion. He enjoined us to "percuss to feel and not to hear." The vibration we received in the pleximeter finger laid flat against the chest was, he said, more important than the sound. You can recognize KVT's progeny from our near-silent percussion; if I percuss audibly, it is only to teach, or to demonstrate, say, to a skeptical brother-in-law or spouse.

For sleuths of the caliber of Leithead or KVT, a diagnosis could be lurking in something as simple as a facial expression. Not the dull and coarse facies of a sluggish thyroid or the masklike expression of Parkinson's disease, which are evident to laypeople, but the risus sardonicus (sardonical smile) of tetanus or the facies latrodectismica (a grimacing, flushed, jaw-clenching, puffy-eyed expression) of a patient affected by the toxin from a black widow spider, or the madonna-like facies and transverse smile of a type of muscular dystrophy.

My final exam at the medical school in Madras included a rigorous clinical test with real patients carefully selected for signs and symptoms of a disease. In America, final-year medical students face no such clinical test. Even for specialists in internal medicine, testing with real patients and live examiners was done away with in the mid-seventies, after it was deemed too subjective. Recently, the powers that be put in place the national Clinical Skills Assessment Exam for final-year American medical students, for which the student has to cough up more than a thousand dollars and travel to one of a couple of centers in the country. In my opinion, and the opinion of many academics I talk to, this exam tests everything but clinical skills. It tests the student's ability to make eye contact, to interact with a person *acting* the role of a patient, to follow the appropriate leads in his fictional story. Does it test whether the student can detect an enlarged liver? Or hear the diastolic sound of heart failure? To get a driver's license or a pilot's license, it is axiomatic that an examiner must watch you drive or fly to confirm you have the skill. Not so in medicine.

I recognize that I am an incurable romantic. I teach bedside skills because I hear the ghosts of Auenbrugger; of the celebrated physician Sir William Osler, who took us out of the classroom a century ago; and of the old horse-and-buggy doctors in South Texas who could divine their patients' maladies by touch, smell, sight, and sound. I hear them say, "Thou shalt not break the chain."

For the past few years in San Antonio, I have spent Wednesday afternoons on "professor's rounds" with six or seven third-year medical students, seeing patients they have worked up. Each week, when I round with a new group, I ask them not to tell me or the other students what the patient's diagnosis is, so that we can see how much the body alone might reveal. The students love these sessions. They often say that this is what they envisioned medicine would be about: time spent in the hallowed space around the patient's bed, time spent with the patient, probing the body for clues. I preach that it is a skill they should cultivate, not to replace technology but to allow them to use technology judiciously and to ask better questions of the tests.

At a recent Wednesday-afternoon session, our patient, an elderly veteran, was thrilled by the attention from the flock of students, particularly their percussing of his chest. "My doctor used to do that when I was a boy," he said with a smile. "He sure knew what he was doing."

Index Case

PERRI KLASS

Because of my extensive training—four years of medical school, three years of pediatric residency, a two-year fellowship in pediatric infectious diseases—and because of my years of experience in practice, I had no trouble at all diagnosing my illness. I knew what was wrong with me, and I knew the technical term for it: I had the pediatric crud. It was winter, and I was seeing sick kids all day long, and now, after a couple of days of congestion and rhinorrhea, a bad cough was developing. It happens every winter, like clockwork.

Now here comes my big confession. I am ashamed to admit that on day one of my bad cough, I started treating myself with antibiotics. Yes, of course, I knew that in all probability I had a viral upper respiratory infection (URI), and I could probably even have named the most likely viruses. And yes, of course, I knew that antibiotics were completely useless in the setting of a viral URI, and I knew that the overuse of antibiotics is a terrible problem in our society, and that the demands of patients with viral illnesses and URIs to be treated with antibiotics need to be met with careful education and explanations—certainly not with unnecessary prescriptions. I knew all that, really I did.

On the other hand, I also knew that in winters past, when my annual pediatric crud dragged into its third or fourth week, I usually ended up taking antibiotics. I would wait until my symptoms qualified to be considered bronchitis, or until a colleague listened to my lungs and heard some crackles; but, in the end, my annual illness would always lead to antibiotics. So since this cough seemed to have gotten so bad so quickly, I reasoned, why not just take the antibiotics right away and see if I could shorten the course? Well, maybe "reasoned" isn't quite the right verb. Let's just say that, more than a little shamefacedly, I treated myself with a five-day course of azithromycin.

It didn't help at all. My cough got worse and worse. I didn't feel too sick otherwise, but I was carrying around a jar of maximum-strength over-the-counter cough medicine, dosing myself whenever I had to see patients, teach, or do anything else that called for conversation. I viewed it as my right and proper punishment for taking unnecessary antibiotics. It never occurred to me to stop seeing patients, of course; nor did it occur to any of my coworkers, I would guess, that perhaps I shouldn't be working. I wasn't really sick, I just had the crud, and we're all wedded to that die-with-your-boots-on ethos whereby you keep on working unless you are sicker than your sickest patients. One day, when I was responsible for hospital rounds, I did ask a colleague whether she thought it might be better to have someone else run over to the hospital and see a couple of newborns—I have this pretty dramatic cough, I said, and I feel a little guilty about coughing in the newborn nursery. My colleague, supremely unimpressed, and much too tight for time herself to fit in an unexpected hospital stop, sensibly suggested that I try a gown, a mask, and gloves.

So, well swathed, I rounded on the babies, and then I went on to work the evening session at the health center, seeing patients. I took the maximum-strength cough medicine and washed my hands scrupulously, and whenever I felt a coughing fit coming on in the presence of a patient, I would make some excuse to leave the room and go cough my head off in the doctors' work area. Then, the colleague who had suggested the gown and mask heard me coughing that very night and remarked that I sounded paroxysmal.

Now, "paroxysmal" is one of those coded medical words. It's like saying a baby seems a little "lethargic," rather than simply tired and clingy and cranky. You say it one way, you mean the baby has a little bug; you say it the other way, you mean do a lumbar puncture. So when she said "paroxysmal," I thought, for the very first time, of pertussis (whooping cough). And once I had started thinking about it, I couldn't get it out of my mind—after all, I had my cough to remind me. So I went to my internist, who thought my lungs sounded fine and that my cough probably just represented a lingering viral illness—and these coughs, she warned me, can last for some time—and that pertussis was highly unlikely. But to allay my anxieties, she sent off a titer (I was more than two weeks into the cough by this point, so it was too late for a culture). And then I went back to seeing patients, and the laboratory misplaced the sample (by filing it under my first name instead of my last, it turned out), and I had to call a friend in Infection Control, who got someone at the lab to take another look, and eventually the sample was found—and guess what? I had pertussis.

I had suddenly become a public health emergency. A pediatrician, seeing children all day, rounding on newborns, the mother of three children at three different schools, the close colleague of who-knows-how-many doctors and nurses and clerical staff. I was phoned or paged by someone from Public Health every day, sometimes several times a day. I sat at my desk making a list of every friend or acquaintance with whom I had been in close contact during my infectious period.

I felt deeply, deeply ashamed. Calling these people, one after another, I felt alternately like Typhoid Mary and the person at the end of the STD partner-notification line. I had exposed them, contaminated them, put them at risk. I urged everyone to take prophylactic antibiotics, to call the doctor immediately if a cough developed. Most of all, though, I felt ashamed before my colleagues and my patients at the health center. I couldn't stand to look at the letter that was going out to the families I had seen during my period of maximal infectiousness: "Your child may have been exposed to a staff member who has pertussis." I did not want to be the doctor who saw any of those families when they came in to get their antibiotics or, if they were coughing, their nasal swabs and their antibiotics. I did not want any of them to know that I was the staff member with pertussis. And to make matters worse, I was still coughing—now not infectious but still coughing pretty dramatically, just in case the local public health emergency had slipped anyone's mind for even a minute.

Some of my anxieties were relatively well grounded in reality. Pertussis, after all, is most dangerous to infants, who account for almost all the hospitalizations and the deaths associated with the disease. And the surveillance data show a steady increase in the rate of disease among infants in the United States between 1980 and 1999—an increase that may be attributable in part to increased transmission from adults.[1] And here I was, one of those adults. We do know that much pertussis disease in adolescents and adults may present as nonspecific or persistent cough, and may therefore go unrecognized.[2] We do not know why the rate of disease in adults should be on the increase, if in fact it is. The confluence of various factors may be to blame: the waning immunity of the vaccinated adolescent and adult population, for instance, and the decreased likelihood that immunity will be boosted by exposure to natural disease.

I was an adult, vaccinated as a child, presumably with waning immunity, which had probably been boosted by exposure to some natural disease during my childhood, forty years ago, and perhaps by the occasional occupational exposure (I can remember at least two occasions during my residency when prophylaxis was prescribed, though I have to confess that, back in those days, when two weeks of erythromycin were required, my compliance was dubious and I probably did not finish either course). Maybe my own waning vaccine-induced immunity finally intersected with a sufficiently infectious exposure—but epidemiologic specu-lation feels different when you yourself are the index case. What I kept picturing were sick babies—individual tiny bodies wracked with coughing fits. There were all the infants I had examined in the clinic, there were the babies in the nursery . . . there was even a friend who had shared a cab with me who had a newborn grandchild, and I imag-ined the chain of risk and exposure stretching far enough to threaten that baby as well.

Of course, I had seen pertussis. I saw a very dramatic case during my residency, in an infant who had deliberately not been vaccinated ("crunchy granola parents," we resi-dents whispered to one another), who was brought into the emergency room looking terrific, but his parents had tape-recorded his coughing spells, telling us they had never heard anything like this. And indeed the spells were terrifying: you listened to the tape, and you could swear the baby was dying of strangulation before your very ears. And at the end of each spell came that terrifying unearthly whoop, as if the baby were possessed by some evil-intentioned spirit of respiratory compromise. Every resident and medical student in the hospital was brought to that baby's room during his hospitalization, and the word was passed: once you hear a real whoop, you'll never forget it (an audio clip is available at www.nejm.org). Well, I had never forgotten it, but adults, by and large, don't whoop, so it had never occurred to me that I might have the same disease as that baby. Some pediatric infectious diseases specialist; some diagnostic whiz kid!

I'm not sure now exactly why I was so ashamed. Presumably, after all, I had contracted pertussis in the line of duty—pediatric infections are an occupational risk and, for all our careful hand washing, if you see sick kids all day long, sometimes some enterprising microorganism makes the jump, through direct contact, through fomite, or through respiratory droplet. It is a professional responsibility, and even a professional point of pride, not to run from the sick but to move toward them and touch them. But there was something about the idea that, instead of helping, I might have gone from day to day and from exam room to exam room doing harm that left me deeply embarrassed. In addition, I was embarrassed that, despite all that training, the word "pertussis" never crossed my mind until someone else listened to my cough with interest and characterized it for me.

There was only one really bright element in those bleak few days, as I huddled over my list of exposed friends, calling them up one after another with the bad news, as I went slinking through the health center imagining resentful looks from nurses and doctors and patients alike: at least I had taken antibiotics, and taken them early. The public health nurse who was assigned to my messy case kept saying it to me on the phone: "Thank God you took those pills!" Because I had started taking azithromycin (which, in Massachusetts, is now a recommended treatment for pertussis) on day one of my cough, I was considered to be noninfectious by day five, so instead of contacting and prophylactically treating about two weeks' worth of patients, we ended up with a relatively short list of children who might have been exposed—and the consolation that even when I saw many of those children, I had been at least partially treated, which might have reduced the risk of transmission. Those babies in the newborn nursery, for example, were not considered to be at risk. And I found myself saying it to my friends, when I called to notify them: "Now, I did take antibiotics right away, but since we spent some time together before I was fully treated, I just wanted to let you know . . ." And as time went on and we failed to uncover any secondary cases that could be traced to me, I kept reminding everyone about that early antibiotic treatment, as if it let me cling to some shreds of doctorly dignity: I had done the right thing, I had used my special knowledge, I had protected those I could protect. In other words, I consoled myself for my irrational sense of shame about having possibly exposed patients to infection with an irrational sense of self-satisfaction about having taken antibiotics for no good reason.

Pertussis may be on the increase in this country, but in many ways it still seems like a disease that does not quite belong to our era. When I had to call people and announce, "I have whooping cough," I felt like a medical curiosity, or the punch line of someone's ironic anecdote: the pediatrician with the rare, vaccine-preventable disease. When the public health officials were calling me, I felt like some other kind of epidemiologic specimen: patient zero, the walking disease-control headache. And through the whole experience, every so often, all my various emotions would disappear into a true and impressive paroxysm of coughing, coughing, and more coughing, as the microbiology and the respiratory pathology took over and left me doubled over, momentarily speechless, and gasping for breath.

Notes

1. M. Tanaka, C. R. Vitek, F. B. Pascual, K. M. Bisgard, J. E. Tate, T. V. Murphy, "Trends in Pertussis Among Infants in the United States, 1980–1999," *Journal of the American Medical Association* 290, no. 22 (2003): 2968–2975.
2. Centers for Disease Control and Prevention, "Pertussis—United States, 1997–2000," *Morbidity and Mortality Weekly Report* 51 (2002): 73–76 (available online at www.cdc.gov/mmwr/PDF/wk/mm5104.pdf).

Resurrectionist

PAULINE W. CHEN

My very first patient had been dead for over a year before I laid hands on her.

It was the mid-1980s, and I had at last made the transition from premedical to full-fledged medical student. That late summer from the window of my dormitory room, I could see the vastness of Lake Michigan dotted with sailboats and the grunting, glistening runners loping along its Chicago shores. Despite this placid view, I rarely looked out my window. I was far too preoccupied with what lay ahead: my classmates and I were about to begin the dissection of a human cadaver.

Prior to that September, the only time I had seen a dead person was at the funeral of my Agong, my maternal grandfather. Agong had grown up on a farm in the backwaters of Taiwan at the turn of the last century. He barely finished high school, but by the time he was middle-aged, Agong owned a jewelry store in one of Taipei's most fashionable districts and had raised five college-educated children. While he grew up speaking Taiwanese, Agong had taught himself Mandarin Chinese and Japanese, languages and dialects as different as German, English, and French.

Agong loved my mother, his firstborn child, and lavished her with that gift of nearly blind parental adoration. As *her* firstborn child, I was in a special position to receive some of those rays of love. Unfortunately though, with my American upbringing I understood Taiwanese but spoke only "Chinglish," a pidgin amalgamation of English and Mandarin Chinese. Moreover, Agong and I had been separated by half a world until he moved permanently to the United States when I was in high school. So while I loved my grandfather, our relationship always remained rather formal.

Agong died in the fall of my sophomore year in college. One weekend, my parents mentioned to me on the phone that he was doing worse and might possibly "not make it." A week later they called again to tell me that he had passed away.

My mother was grief-stricken. She became consumed by guilt and remorse, feelings that I would later learn often plague relatives of the recently dead. For my part, while I did mourn Agong's death, I was unsure how to cope with this phase of life or with my mother's overwhelming grief. I had not been witness to his actual dying, and seeing my grandfather alive during one visit and lying dead in a casket the next made his death unreal to me. The funeral was not particularly long, but the parade of mourners dressed in black and my own uneasy feelings seemed to last forever.

I was surprised by how *un*-lifelike Agong looked lying in the casket. Despite all the efforts of the mortician, the figure in the coffin simply looked like a model of Agong, like a wax figure from Madame Tussauds's famous museum. His face and body as I had known them were gone. Even his nose, famous in our family for its Jimmy Durante profile, had changed; the nostrils looked less fleshy and even droopy, like a once majestic sail that had lost its wind.

The fact that even the professionals with all their makeup and tricks could not re-create my grandfather's likeness only served to emphasize that he was really dead and gone from our lives. That funeral, the telephone call from my parents announcing my grandfather's passing, and the memories of my mother's grieving were the most direct experiences with death that I had prior to medical school.

The majority of my 170 medical school classmates were no more experienced than I, and our first real exposure to death would be that semester in the human anatomy course. While one student had worked in a hospital morgue during college and another had worked in an Illinois meatpacking plant (subsequently becoming a strict vegetarian), those two classmates were the rare exception. Instead, the summer before starting medical school most of us privately dreaded and fretted about dissecting a human being.

During my medical school orientation week, I was finally able to share my dissection fears with others who harbored the same uneasiness. Anatomy quickly became a major topic of discussion at social events. The classmate who had worked in a morgue was a prime source of information for the rest of us. I kept wondering if the cadavers looked alive or like wax figures. I secretly hoped that they would look at least as unreal as my grandfather had, believing that the less they looked like the living, the easier dissecting would be. We asked the second-year medical students about their experience the previous year. "Wear your old T-shirts and jeans," they said, sipping their drinks nonchalantly at receptions for the new initiates. "You'll want to throw out those clothes at the end of the semester because they'll just reek." Holding on to their words, I replayed their cavalier responses in my mind. What smell would cling to our clothes? Death?

From the moment I had begun contemplating this career path some fifteen years earlier, I knew that I would want to use my profession to help people. Most of my classmates were no different. We were an odd group, idealistic but intensely obsessive and competitive enough to have survived the grueling premedical curriculum. While a few of us might have harbored goals of financial security or visions of a certain lifestyle, we were for the most part determined to learn how to save lives.

What many of us did not realize was that despite those dreams, our profession would require us to live among the dying. Death, more than life, would become the constant in our lives.

The dissection of the human body had fascinated me since I was seven years old. I had some idea back then that I might want to become a doctor. At the time my Agong had just been diagnosed with a brain tumor, and my mother took my younger sister and me back to Taiwan for the summer to be with him. The diagnosis, the operation, and the neurologic deficits resulting from the removal of a part of my grandfather's brain would eventually color the rest of my grandparents' lives together. Nonetheless, at the time I was enthralled by the way his neurosurgeon comforted my grandmother and family. He was a big, bald Taiwanese man, with a round face, hands like bear paws, and a demeanor that was at once humble and confident. When he came out to the waiting room to an audience of anxious family members, his words—"I got it all out"—fell on us like a great light from the heavens. That experience convinced me that medicine was the work of gods.

An aunt who was in medical school at the time heard about my interest and offered to take me to her anatomy lab. I was fascinated by the idea that there might be secrets about life and death lurking there. At that age I already had come to believe that dissection was the greatest event that separated physicians from the rest of us. To be able to stomach such an experience, I thought, would prove my mettle, and to sneak a peek into the inner workings of a body—a dead body, no less—would put me in a league beyond any other second-grader I knew. My parents, however, quickly vetoed the idea, fearing that such a close-up and possibly gruesome experience might scar me permanently.

Like all initiation rites, the dissection of the human cadaver poses several obstacles to the neophyte. First, the new medical student has to memorize a vast array of anatomical facts. Such rote memorization can be mindnumbingly dull, and the overwhelming amount of information makes the task seem Sisyphean. One of my college mentors, a brilliant psychiatrist and anthropologist, counseled me before I started. He had completed medical school some twenty years earlier. "It's like memorizing a telephone book," he said. "You just have to get through it."

Memorization, however, is probably the easiest obstacle to surmount, and it has until recently been the only focus of medical schools. The more difficult, and often unspoken, obstacle for medical students is accepting death and the violation of the human body. In the human anatomy course, cadavers are laid before fledgling physicians, and the familiarity of their form reminds us that each lived lives not unlike our own. For those of us who wince from simple paper cuts, running a scalpel against skin and definitively dividing the essential structures that once powered a fellow human are acts that require a leap of faith. While all premedical students fully expect to perform a human cadaver dissection in medical school, the expectation hardly tempers the brutal reality.

Aspiring physicians face death directly in the form of the cadaver. And then they tear it apart. Each detail of the cadaver—every bone, nerve, blood vessel, and muscle—

passes from the world of the unknown into the realm of the familiar. Every cavity is probed, every groove explored, and every crevice pulled apart. In knowing the cadaver in such intimate detail, we believe that we are acquiring the knowledge to overcome death.

To complete the initiation rite successfully, however, we need to learn to separate our emotional self from our scientific self; we must view this dead human body not as "one of us" but as "one of them," a medical case to be understood but not embraced. This ability to distance the self, I was to learn later, would be called upon again and again in my medical training. It was as if such separation would provide me with a greater sense of objectivity, a modicum of strength, and thus an enhanced ability to care for my patients. But this first lesson in disengaging from the personal was the most radical: it required suppressing the fundamental and very human fear of death.

My medical school, not entirely unaware of the anxiety we harbored, did make some attempts to lessen the impact of working with a cadaver. We spent a week in lectures preparing for the first day of dissection. While none of these lectures directly addressed our mounting anxieties, they did give us the tools we needed to begin to detach ourselves emotionally from the experience. One of our first anatomic lessons was on vocabulary used to describe the body. These words, so different from our usual descriptive terms, would serve as directions on the map of the human body. We learned the difference between "distal" and "proximal," "abduct" and "adduct," "transverse" and "sagittal." We learned that "left" and "right" no longer referred to our left and right but to the patient's.

The day before our first dissection lab, we toured the laboratory facilities. There were eleven rooms connected by a long hallway, and each room had four large stone lab benches with sinks and enough workspace for four students. A large enclosed cavity within the lab benches held a sliding metal bed not unlike the metal beds used by coroners or pathologists. These cavities would be where our cadavers would be stored. We would spend every weekday afternoon for the next twelve weeks in these rooms, and all of us, either in small groups or alone, would spend many of our free hours there trying to memorize the minutiae from each cadaver.

Formaldehyde, the preservative used for cadavers, has an unmistakable odor—sharp, rancid, piercing—like the olfactory version of a high-pitched shriek. The faint smell of formaldehyde present in each of the eleven rooms was left over from years past, as the cadavers for our class had not yet arrived. Over the years the smell had managed to work its way into the rooms' marble and concrete, lingering and reminding us of our place in the school's history.

Our professor was not the wizened sage I had always envisioned would take me through this rite. Instead, he was just a few years out from his own graduate work in physical anthropology and anatomy. His youth and strong Hoosier twang demystified the whole ritual and made many of us more relaxed. He informed us of the overwhelming power of the scent of formaldehyde and reminded us that the smell would permeate our gloved hands, clothes, and hair. Indeed, I would soon discover that it would be strange eating with my hands that semester. While tasting some chicken wings at a reception later that fall, I realized that the smell of the cadavers from my fingers was mingling with the taste of barbecued chicken in my mouth. "Lemon dishwashing detergent helps get rid of the smell," our professor advised us the afternoon before we were to embark on our dissections. That night each of us pulled out clothes that we were willing to toss at the end of three months—frayed jeans, "borrowed" hospital scrubs, and T-shirts with high school emblems—and there was a run on lemon dishwashing detergent at the local grocery stores.

The next afternoon an intensified odor assaulted each of us as we entered the labs; overnight, the laboratory technicians had placed fresh cadavers in their respective stone enclaves. For that afternoon's work I had replaced my contact lenses, susceptible to the fumes of formaldehyde, with my chunky glasses, and I remember being mildly surprised by how many of my fellow classmates were as blind as I. All of us had also carefully put on thin yellow paper masks, more to blunt the penetrating formaldehyde than to protect ourselves from any biohazards. Over the weeks, as we became more absorbed in our work, we eventually neglected to wear these flimsy barriers. Some of us even occasionally forgot to put on our gloves.

The class was divided alphabetically into groups of four students, and each group was assigned to a cadaver. These groupings were used over and over again during the next two years whenever our education required more intimate instruction. With the same three classmates, we clumsily attempted to draw blood, learned to do pelvic exams, and performed our first rectal exams on patients. Most notably, however, we dissected together in anatomy lab.

I worked with three other women. Mary was from California, the daughter of a family practitioner and the middle child in a large Irish-Italian Catholic family. She was preternaturally calm, a characteristic that would give her an outstanding bedside manner, and she eventually followed in her father's footsteps. Peg was from Chicago. She was the most reticent of the four but made up for her shyness with a generous spirit and a sharp, dry wit that helped give the rest of us perspective during more difficult times. She later became a pediatrician. The third woman, Lara, was the youngest and the most boisterous of the four of us. The daughter of immigrants, she was born and raised in Chicago and now practices pediatrics in that city. I was from New England and set at the time on becoming a psychiatrist or geriatrician and pursuing an academic career in medical anthropology. However, as gruesome as it all seemed to me that first week, the experience of the cadaver dissection— the concise and efficient beauty of human anatomy, the pleasure of using my hands as an extension of my mind, and the spirit of teamwork—became the foundation of my decision to become a surgeon.

On that first day I unlatched the door on the side of our stone lab bench and gently slid the metal bed out of the inner compartment. All the cadavers were sheathed in white plastic body bags. Some bags were large; others were smaller. There was no question, however, given the frozen forms, what was within these zippered shrouds. Several provisions had been made by the medical school to decrease the shock of starting our work. The lab technicians had placed all the bodies facedown so that we could see only the back of their head. We started our daily dissections with the arms and legs, and our cadavers' faces were kept covered until the final two weeks of the course. Those who organized our anatomy course believed that such a progression would be a gentler introduction to working on a dead human being.

We learned anatomic principles, dissection techniques, and ways to hold the dissecting instruments with greater precision. We learned that in medicine, "tweezers" were called "forceps," and those who fancied a future career in surgery used the more specialized jargon, "pickups." We learned to change blades efficiently on a scalpel without ever touching the blade's sharp edge, to hold the scalpel like a pencil for finer work, and to grasp it with the tips of four fingers and the thumb apposed, as if holding a violin bow, for more dramatic slices and cuts. We began to manipulate scissors with the thumb and fourth finger, as surgeons do, not the thumb and index finger as we had once learned in nursery school. "Using the fourth finger allows the index finger to rest on the joint of the scissors and gives greater control," stated one of the teaching assistants, a fourth-year medical student planning on a surgical career. Hairdressers everywhere, I would later note, hold scissors in a similar fashion.

The only information that we had on our cadavers was a card attached to the bag indicating their gender and approximate age at death. My cadaver was a woman who had died at seventy-two. Other than those two pieces of information, there was nothing else: no name, no address, no story. It was unsettling to be presented with so little history, and it became more so as we allowed ourselves to become intimately familiar with every detail of these bodies. My lab partners and I would know our cadaver's body better than any patient we would ever take care of; yet in her book of life, we were to begin with the epilogue and attempt to read backward.

Despite all the precautions taken by my medical school, my cadaver hardly remained an impersonal corpse with anonymous extremities. I remember unzipping the white bag that held her and being surprised by her thin arms. Her fingers were long and slender, with delicate, pointed tips; her nails had been filed into fine ovals and painted with coral nail polish. It was probably time for another manicure, as just above her neatly maintained cuticles were slender little half-moons of bare pink nail. While the skin around her forearm seemed to wrap tightly around her muscles, the skin on her upper arm was looser. It was wrinkled and hardened, like old leather. I figured that the hardening must have been from the time spent in a vat of formaldehyde.

My lab partners and I took scalpels to the skin of our cadaver, making long incisions along the length of the hand and forearm. In so interrupting the tension of the skin, we released the dermal tissue and muscles from their epidermal cocoons. We then gently stripped and separated that tissue with fine scissors and forceps, traveling along the axes of the vessels and nerves. Moving our cadaver's arm, now free of any skin covering or sinewy attachments, we saw the muscles function with each action and wondered how much more animated they might have been in life.

Aspects of that life were apparent from our cadaver's slender arms. She had loved the sun; the tanned background of her skin betrayed the jewelry that had once adorned her. On her left fourth finger I could see the white imprint of a wedding band. On her wrist I could make out the pale outline of a watch, probably one of those fine old-lady watches with the delicate chain across the latch for security. As we dissected into her hand, encountering the small muscles— flexor pollicis longus, abductor pollicis brevis—I could imagine how each of these bundles of tissue once worked in her hands. The pink flesh, now a grayish red in death, would have contracted, each fiber shortening and swelling with the exertion, the muscle strands pulling on their attachments to her fingers, flexing the fingers around the hand of her husband or the brush she held to her hair.

Trying to memorize the Latin names with no intrinsic meaning to me, I would think of my cadaver's muscles and then imagine my own muscles while waving my arms and legs in front of the bathroom mirror. *Brachioradialis,* I would say to myself as I rotated my forearm and imagined my cadaver doing the same. *Sartorius,* I would think as I sat on a chair and crossed a leg over the opposite knee, imagining this graceful and delicate muscle in my cadaver's thigh and the Roman tailors who gave it its name. The laboratory experience we were struggling with in the afternoons would reinforce, then and forever, the didactic anatomy lectures we heard in the mornings; and to this day, I see my cadaver's body when I envision human anatomy.

We spent two weeks dissecting the arms and legs and began the third week of anatomy with our first exam. During the written portion I spied classmates waving their arms and legs around to jog their memories; they, too, had danced in front of their mirrors. After the written exam we took the practical portion of the test in the laboratories. At various stations our professor displayed dissections from class cadavers with plastic question marks pinned to different structures. The cadavers had been covered so well, except for the vessel or nerve or muscle in question, that it was difficult to figure out what was an arm or a forearm, a leg or a thigh. A timer in the labs went off every two minutes, and as the alarm sounded, each of us scrambled to the next station and struggled to make sense of the disconnected body parts.

In the midst of these cadaveric displays I spied those slender fingers with the coral nail polish and felt a wave of pride. I was pleased with the meticulous work my lab group had done and proud of the beauty of our cadaver's anatomy.

During those early weeks some of my classmates and I began to have dreams about anatomy lab. Some had peaceful dreams in which they held hands with their cadavers or shared a meal. Others were less romantic or downright frightening. My dream, likely fueled by a childhood appreciation of Edgar Allan Poe, remains vivid in my memory. I find myself alone in the laboratory, pacing the hall. The doors of the supply closets that line the hallway swing open suddenly, and cadavers partially dissected and exhibiting signs of putrefaction hang on hooks in each closet. As I try to run away, the closet doors keep opening and closing. Afraid that one of the cadavers will fall on me, I frantically try to escape; but a relentless echoing heartbeat pursues me, growing louder as I run down the hallway.

That morning I woke up exhausted. After a few minutes I realized that the heartbeats I had heard were the reverberations of my own pulse pounding in my ears.

As the weeks passed many of my classmates resorted to black humor. Medical versions of urban legends made the rounds of our laboratories, as they did in medical schools throughout the country. One story was of a medical student who stole a hand and took it to a bar for a variant of the "can you lend me a hand" visual gag. Another story took place at a stadium's urinals with a couple of men, a male medical student, and another stolen anatomic part. One classic legend, probably passed among medical students for generations, had the medical student "friend of a friend" completing dissection on the entire body, only to find upon uncovering the cadaver's face that she had been dissecting her uncle.

Some of my fellow students became increasingly dependent on humor of any kind to lighten the mood in the laboratories and to ease personal anxieties. One group of students brought recordings of old television show theme songs to play while dissecting. Another student adopted the ritual of coming around to each of the four tables in our lab room and playing his air guitar at the beginning of each dissection period. For a while it seemed as if no afternoon could go by without Ben first jamming on that guitar, his thin long face contorted as he lip-synched some classic hard-rock tune playing in his head. Midway through that first semester, however, he and his air guitar suddenly disappeared; Ben had quit medical school.

The daily confrontation with a dead body, the first stranger's body that medical students may have ever examined so closely, marks a point of high anxiety in medical education. Ruth Richardson, in her classic book *Death, Dissection, and the Destitute,* writes, "[D]issection requires in its practitioners the effective suspension or suppression of many normal physical and emotional responses to the willful mutilation of the body of another human being." Traditionally medical schools have rarely addressed such psychological concerns; instead educators have only acknowledged the difficulty of mastering the detailed anatomic knowledge. Taking the cues from their teachers, medical students learn to deny their own feelings, depersonalizing the dissection experience and objectifying their cadaver. They strip away the cadaver's humanity, and soon enough they are dissecting not another human being but "the leg" or "the arm."

There are other not-so-subtle clues that reveal the psychological impact of the experience. The frequent cadaver dreams show how profoundly the experience affects the psyche. The use of black humor allows students to deny the significance of any emotional strain. The medical urban legends allow one to hear about someone else's more horrifying experience and thus put one's own experience in a lesser, and therefore more easily palatable, position. At times the denial becomes so great that young medical students are unable to express even their grief. When their emotions are finally released, the manifestations are strangely inappropriate. Ellen Lerner Rothman, M.D., writes in her memoir of her four years at Harvard Medical School:

> At times, it felt as if death were everywhere. In anatomy lab, we finally uncovered the facial shroud and opened the skull to dissect the brain, and that was okay. I talked to a patient who had nearly died the previous evening and would certainly die within the next months, and that was okay. I came home, and my goldfish had died, and that wasn't okay. I sobbed for half an hour.

Even medical students chosen for their humanitarian qualities and selected from a huge pool of applicants may have their generous impulses profoundly suppressed by their medical education. Some students misinterpret their painful reactions to the dissection process as abnormal and abort their budding medical careers, incorrectly assuming that they have entered the wrong profession.

There are experts in medical education who theorize that the dysfunctional coping mechanisms traditionally used by medical students in their anatomy courses can lead to inappropriately unsympathetic bedside manners. To encourage the development of more effective and desirable attitudes, medical schools have begun to broaden the human anatomy curriculum and have taken steps to mitigate the emotional difficulties. For example, more schools are now holding memorial services for the cadavers at the end of the anatomy course, providing students with an opportunity to express their emotions and gratitude. During these ceremonies, students perform musical pieces and read poems and essays they have written about their cadavers. Some schools have incorporated death-and-dying education into the human anatomy curriculum, drawing on the humanities to generate discussion in small groups and encouraging students to use writing and the fine arts to express their emotions. Still others, plagued by a perpetual shortage of cadavers donated for science, contemplate eliminating dissection altogether, limiting anatomy, and perhaps the student's first encounter with a patient, to a computer-generated experience.

Over the course of the next week our class dissections centered on the perineal and inguinal, or groin, areas. The layers of muscle and fascia around the rectum, vagina, penis, urethra, and groin overlap and undulate in confusing ways. Despite the careful dissection work on our cadavers, many of us remained frustrated. In fact, it was not until my next-to-last year of surgical residency that I fully understood the many layers and folds of tissue encountered in an inguinal hernia repair.

That fall my classmates and I brought our anatomy texts to the library, the conference rooms, the cafeteria, and the subways and stared at the pictures, trying to commit all the parts to memory. A German anatomy atlas became particularly popular during this segment of our course. Instead of paintings or drawings, this book featured photographs of actual cadaveric dissections. Despite the fact that all the named parts looked ragged from preservation and were of an indistinct beige or gray, some of us believed that these books would help us on exams. On full display wherever we were studying, these atlases would be flipped open to photographs of dissected, spread-eagled, cadaveric male and female genitalia. One classmate realized she had become hardened to these depictions when she looked up from her anatomy books and noticed other passengers on her train commute home moving silently away from her.

Male cadavers were rare that year, so we all crowded around the lab groups who had males to watch the dissection of the male external genitalia. One student read from the *Gray's Anatomy* lab instruction book, the bible of anatomic dissections, while another performed the necessary incisions and maneuvers. It was usually the women who held the scalpel during this part of the dissection. I watched my male classmates wince and shift uncomfortably; there were some areas of the body where we could not, try as we may, separate our own feelings from the science of discovery.

The final maneuver of this section of anatomy would, according to our professor, "bring all the concepts together visually." *Divide the pelvis sagittally,* our *Gray's Anatomy* lab instruction book directed. That afternoon in the laboratories we passed around an electric saw similar to the one my father used for carpentry at home. My lab partners were not sure that we understood what we had read. To our disbelief, we did: we would need to bring the saw down the middle of our cadaver's pelvis and divide it. While this step did indeed expose pelvic anatomy in a way that no other dissection would, I could not bring myself to take the saw to our cadaver. Even after having filleted her arms and legs in previous weeks, I had difficulty with the idea of *sawing* a part of her in two. Realizing that three of us could not do it, Mary, the calm one who would become a family physician, took the saw in hand. She closed her eyes for a moment and then drew the spinning blade down from the center of the symphysis pubis to the strip of flesh between the buttock cheeks. Our cadaver's pelvis, now split, fell apart, the legs turning outward like those of a dancer in the first position. Mary turned off the saw, handed it to the next group of waiting students, and remained silent for the rest of the afternoon.

Since medical school, I have loved gazing at historical lithographs of human anatomy. Tucked away in ancient book stacks in medical libraries, sold in overstocked antiquarian bookstores, or displayed in stands along the Seine in Paris, the pictures are not always anatomically correct, but they are always amusing for their profusion of detail and over-the-top quality. The ones from the Renaissance are often accessorized with ornate calligraphy, the tails of letters curling coyly around the borders. The cadavers are artfully posed, as if about to give a lecture or smell a flower, seemingly unconcerned that their innards are hanging out on full display.

Despite the existence of such lithographs for centuries, public acceptance of human cadaver dissection as a part of medical education is a fairly recent phenomenon. For much of their history, anatomists and physicians worked illegally and surreptitiously, lying, cheating, stealing, and even murdering to further their academic cause. The Council of Tours openly prohibited human dissection in 1163. While their edict was directed more at the practice of dismembering and boiling the remains of dead Crusaders for shipment home, the early Christian beliefs regarding postmortem manipulations were clearly reflected in this decree. After all, the resurrection of the body would be impossible if it had been dissected and therefore desecrated.

During the Renaissance there was a surge of interest in

anatomy. Leonardo da Vinci, for example, studied human anatomy in great detail. In 1510 Leonardo completed work that displayed the parallels between human and animal musculature, but his drawings remained unpublished during his lifetime. Andreas Vesalius, the acknowledged father of modern anatomy, performed his own cadaveric dissections and published the seven-volume masterpiece *De Humani Corporis Fabrica* in 1543. His meticulously accurate work revealed that earlier, previously accepted classical authorities such as Galen had been incorrect. Because of religious taboos, the classical anatomists had based their human portraits on animal anatomy.

After the Protestant Reformation in the sixteenth century, London's Royal College of Physicians received the legal authority to dissect human cadavers, but their corpses were limited to those of hanged felons. Dissections at the time were seen as the ultimate punishment for criminals, far worse than a death sentence alone. Even with the corpses of felons, however, the English medical community remained short of cadavers; and surgeons and anatomists resorted to purchasing bodies from grave robbers or "resurrectionists," individuals who exhumed the recently deceased from their graves.

During the nineteenth century Edinburgh was the center of research in anatomy, and Dr. Robert Knox attracted crowds of five hundred or more to his anatomy lectures. The number of aspiring physicians entering the specialty of surgery was also increasing because of the growing respect and honor accorded this profession. The medical school's anatomy and surgery course lasted sixteen months, and students were required to dissect a minimum of three corpses in order to become licensed surgeons. All of these factors further taxed the limited supply of cadavers.

Despite his illustrious reputation, Knox was believed to have remedied this shortage by purchasing bodies from two resurrectionists, William Burke and William Hare. While Burke and Hare did steal corpses from graveyards, they became infamous for having murdered as many as sixteen people in order to sell the bodies. Given the lack of an adequate tissue fixative and ensuing problems of decay, anatomists at the time preferred "fresher" corpses, and the corpses from Burke and Hare were among the most desirable. The two men had devised a technique of asphyxiation that left the cadaver relatively free of any signs of violence. This technique came to be called "burking," a term that eventually worked its way into colloquial English because of the magnitude of the ensuing scandal.

In 1829 Burke was found guilty of murder. His partner, Hare, escaped the death sentence by giving evidence against Burke during the trial. Burke was hanged in front of thirty thousand people, and his body was, rather appropriately, made the subject of a public dissection. His death mask and a wallet made from his tanned skin remain on display at the Anatomy Museum of the Royal College of Surgeons in Edinburgh. As for Dr. Knox, investigators were never able to prove his role in the multiple burkings, but suspicion was so high that the previously esteemed professor was driven out of Edinburgh amid a public frenzy.

In response to the outcry and a subsequent case of burking in 1831, London passed the Warburton Anatomy Act of 1832, which ended the use of dissection as a punishment for murder and gave anatomists unlimited access to unclaimed pauper bodies from workhouses and hospitals. This law ultimately increased the supply of corpses, but many believed that it also transferred the worst punishment for criminals over to the indigent.

In the New World the same social and political forces were at work. While human cadaver dissections took place in America as early as 1638, the demand for cadaver sources began to increase in 1745, when the first formal course in anatomy was offered at the University of Pennsylvania. The only cadavers available legally, however, were the bodies of executed criminals; dissection was used as a form of supra-capital punishment, just as in England. In 1784, for example, to discourage dueling, a Massachusetts law proclaimed that a slain duelist could be either buried without a coffin in a public place and with a stake driven through his body, or given to a surgeon for dissection. Six years later federal judges gained the right to add dissection to the death sentence for murder.

When American medical schools began proliferating in the early nineteenth century, grave robbing became rampant as the demand for cadavers rose. The public became enraged by these acts of desecration and took to the streets in almost a dozen riots between 1765 and 1852. In April 1788, for example, children playing on the streets peered through the windows of the Society of the Hospital of the City of New York and saw medical students dissecting human cadavers. Their parents became outraged when they investigated and saw the dissected corpses. One child's father even discovered that his late wife's corpse, robbed from the grave, was among the dissected. A mob of five thousand stormed the hospital and the jail where several of the doctors had fled to take refuge. A three-day riot ensued, the laboratory was burned down, and seven rioters were killed. The militia finally dispersed the crowd by firing muskets. In response to these riots, New York passed a law in 1789 that allowed doctors to obtain human cadavers without resorting to body snatching.

By the end of the nineteenth century most states had

passed laws that allowed medical schools to obtain un-claimed bodies. The impetus for these laws came in 1878, when U.S. Senator John Scott Harrison, the son of President William Henry Harrison and father of President Benjamin Harrison, died and was buried in Ohio. Soon after Senator Harrison's funeral, his son and nephew received word that the body of a family friend, William Devin, had been stolen from its grave and taken to the Medical College of Ohio. The two men went to the anatomy laboratory of the medical school to look for Devin. Instead, they found the body of Senator Harrison about to undergo dissection.

By 1968 all fifty states had adopted the Uniform Ana-tomical Gift Act. This act ensures that a donor can bequeath his or her body to medical science and education. Since then medical schools have decreased the number of unclaimed bodies used, and the majority of cadavers studied now are the result of conscious and thoughtful decisions made by individuals prior to death. Nonetheless, the ongoing need for bodies and anatomic parts has created latter-day resur-rectionists. Two recent cases of body parts being sold—by employees at a California medical school and by a dentist and funeral home director in New York—remind us of nightmares rooted in our collective history.

Despite the difficult history of anatomy, the act of dis-secting a human cadaver—of feeling and seeing and holding the human body and its parts—remains fundamental to medical education. For physicians, the experience remains one of the most transformative in their early professional lives.

We moved next in our anatomic journey to the torso. To acclimate our tender hearts to the grisly task, our teachers

instructed us to start with the more impersonal back muscles. With fresh blades on our scalpels, we sliced through
and peeled away the skin and subcutaneous layers, exposing
the pale reddish-brown muscle fibers. The group across
from us had a hulking male cadaver who had died in the
prime of life. The muscles on his back were large and developed and reminded me of the big chunks of meat I had seen
in the butcher's section of the local supermarket. From that
point on in my life, I had little enthusiasm for eating red
meat; it never tasted the same again.

In contrast, my cadaver had little if any muscular development, and I wondered if my own scrawny back was like
hers. Compared to the other cadavers, particularly the
males, my cadaver's back muscles seemed barely large
enough to have once held her torso erect. Some of her muscular structures were so small that I felt as if I were imagining rather than really seeing the muscles I had read about in
my anatomy instruction book. While the larger straps of
muscle on my classmates' cadavers were easier to study, I felt
possessive of my cadaver and became almost defensive about
the tiny strings of tissue that crossed her spine and rib cage.

After dissecting these muscles, we turned our cadavers
on their backs and began work on the chest. My three female
lab partners and I dissected the breasts particularly gently.
We had read about Cooper's ligaments, strings of nearly
invisible tissue that suspend the glands, and the complicated
ductal system. Much to our dismay, however, we found that
the inner tissue of the breast was yellow and globular, not
that dissimilar from the fat that we found in other parts of
the body. The special ducts and glands that made milk for
babies looked just like chicken fat with white, tenuous, con-
nective tissue strings interspersed. It all appeared bland and
nondescript.

We peeled away the rest of the skin and subcutaneous tissue to expose the muscles of the chest. The pectoralis major and the pectoralis minor were splayed like magnificent fans across each side. Underneath, the breastbone connected the two halves of the thorax like the hinge on a treasure chest, each rib's tendinous connection like a joint of that hinge. We used another kind of electric saw to perform a median sternotomy, a maneuver that would divide the breastbone along its length, as surgeons do during cardiac operations. Using our index fingers in a technique appropriately referred to as "blunt dissection," we cleared two small spaces just beneath the top and bottom of the sternum; these were the starting and finishing points for our little jigsaw. I revved up the humming motor of the saw, inserted its tip into the divot between our cadaver's collarbones, and drew the vibrating blade along the length of the sternum.

My lab partners and I pulled apart each side of the split breastbone. Underneath we found a pale sac, the pericardium, that enveloped our cadaver's heart. I divided the sac with dissection scissors, thumb and fourth finger in the rings of the instrument. Underneath, a ball of muscle just barely the size of my fist squatted like a bulldog guarding a house. We removed the heart, cutting across its great vessels with large scissors similar to sewing shears, and then spent the rest of the day examining its anatomy. We dissected out the paperlike mitral valve, so named because its two leaflets resemble the pope's miter. Sitting between the left atrium and the left ventricle, the mitral valve is tethered around its periphery by strands of muscle that look like the cords on a parachute. We dissected out the coronary arteries, each barely larger than a sharpened pencil tip. When these arteries are blocked, essential oxygen cannot reach the heart, and this ischemia can result in the death of heart muscle, otherwise known as a myocardial infarction or a heart attack. I stared at these crucial tiny vessels, amazed that people did not suffer heart attacks any earlier in life.

On each side of the now empty pericardium were the lungs, deflated and still. According to our textbooks, each lung was made up of hundreds of millions of microscopic biological balloons called alveoli. Areas that were still inflated were particularly soft, almost velvety. A finger pressed into them left a small glistening depression and made a quiet wet sound, like the one made by a foot on the muddy banks of a pond. Our cadaver's lungs were black and speckled with soot. Initially I thought that the formaldehyde had discolored them, but when I saw the other cadavers' chests—our strapping neighbor's lungs were full and pink— I realized that our cadaver had had a lifetime of cigarettes and some tough city living.

We removed the lungs, cutting across the tubes and vessels that once supplied air and blood. The thoracic cavity, with puddles of formaldehyde settled on the dependent back side, now looked like an emptied, darkened fishbowl. From within we could follow several nerves that extended across the chest wall. The phrenic nerve, whose tiny electrical pulses innervate the muscular diaphragm, seemed hardly like the miserable perpetrator of intractable hiccoughs, but more like a long strand of spaghetti al dente. The imposing aortic arch, that magnificent muscular artery that once carried the oxygenated blood with a great kick from the heart, curved elegantly up toward the brain and then down again toward the abdomen; I could imagine blood jetting from its cavernous hollow into meandering and progressively smaller arteries throughout the body.

We moved downward to the abdomen. We incised the skin, went through the subcutaneous fat, and then dissected out the abdominal wall muscles. Our cadaver's belly was flat, but her abdominal wall hung strangely, given her fine bone structure. There was a looseness to her belly's skin and musculature, as if it had once been round and full, and the muscles here were atrophied and stringy. An old surgical incision traveled in a fine long line from her breastbone to her pubis and distorted the tiny opening in her abdominal wall that would have been her navel.

Once inside her abdominal cavity, we noticed that her intestines seemed oddly tangled. Other cadavers had bowels that were easily manipulated and could slide around freely, as they might have during peristalsis and digestion. My three lab partners and I found ourselves in a maze of bowel loops with no discernible beginning or end. We repeated the mantra of anatomic dissections: *Go from the known to the unknown.* Normally, there is enough consistency in human anatomy that one can recognize newly dissected structures by following the lines of those already identified. We each took a turn trying to make sense of the matted intestines, but the instructions of the anatomy textbook—*Follow the small intestine down to the terminal ileum where you will find the appendix*—confused us even more.

Unlike her orderly arms, back, and chest, our cadaver's abdomen was in disarray. She had no gallbladder. Her omentum, the fatty bib that usually covers the bowels, was gone. Adhesions, scar tissue, distorted her intra-abdominal anatomy, coalescing the delicate individual organs into a big, ugly block.

It was obvious that our cadaver had had surgery of some kind, but what operation could have left her abdominal contents so decimated? My lab partners and I finally went to look at our classmates' cadavers, where the anatomy was more clearly discernible. Each of us was silently disappointed, feeling as if our cadaver had betrayed us and kept the secrets of abdominal anatomy hidden from our probing hands and minds.

By the eighth week of anatomy class, we had dissected our way down to the pelvis. I was immensely curious about the uterus and ovaries. I wanted to see and feel them. What were the organs that held babies and created menstrual periods really like? I remembered my sixth-grade Family Life teacher, Miss Goodwin, explaining menstruation and ovulation. As one of the youngest teachers in my elementary school, Joanna Goodwin had likely been unwillingly corralled into the job of teaching sex education to fifty prepubescent girls. Nonetheless, she managed to be both creative and entertaining. When asked to describe the uterus and ovaries, Miss Goodwin paused momentarily from her fast-paced presentation. Finally, she held both arms up in the air and placed balled-up newspaper in each hand. "Do you see?" she asked us. "My body is the uterus, my arms are the fallopian tubes, and the newspapers are the ovaries."

I half expected to see Miss Goodwin in our cadaver's pelvis, her arms outstretched and her hands grasping two crumpled balls of newspaper. As we delved deeper, my lab partners and I began instead to find balls of hardened tissue. Eager to see the female reproductive organs, we proclaimed the first two balls to be the ovaries. Our cadaver, however, kept bringing forth more balls of tissue, some as small as marbles, others as big as limes. The numerous balls were stuck together, stuck to intestine, stuck to her inner pelvic wall. Some were smooth, but many were like rocks with craggy faces. We called our professor over. He peered into our cadaver's abdominal cavity. "Oh my," he said. "I think she had ovarian cancer."

The ovaries that produced the estrogen that gave our

cadaver the feminine features and qualities she cared for so dearly were the very organs that would put an end to her life. At one unknown moment in her life, one of her ovarian cells contorted and mutated and then began to reproduce with unchecked fervor. The anomalous ovarian tissue grew and infiltrated her intestines, causing them to mat together and obstruct. The cancerous tissue produced fluid, ascites, in her belly, which caused the once flat waistline to stretch and bloat and robbed our cadaver of her delicate figure. In death, in that vat of formaldehyde, her ascites had disappeared, so now her stretched abdominal wall hung loosely over her slender frame. The chemotherapy she received in an attempt to hold on to life had left her scalp bare except for a few soft, downy strands. The tumor that had greedily robbed her body of nutrients in its maniacal race to grow had left our cadaver wasted and thin, so that even her back muscles had degenerated into a few measly strings.

Our classmates took a particular interest in the findings in our cadaver's abdomen. As physicians who are meant to cure the ill, we are lifelong students not of the normal but of the abnormal, the anomalies and curiosities of human physiology. Here was a chance to see ovarian cancer in the flesh; for some students it would be their only chance to see the end stages of this disease process. During that long afternoon the anatomy instructors pointed out the irregular agglomerations of tumor in our group's cadaver, and our classmates wandered by and marveled at her intra-abdominal contents. In many ways this scene was a preview of our future as clinicians, when we would, in large groups on clinical rounds, visit living patients. Our preoccupation as medical students with seeing and touching abnormal findings in cadavers already reflected this voyeuristic aspect of our art. Even at the beginning of our schooling, we realized that great clinicians are not just born; they are trained.

By the time my lab partners and I finally uncovered our cadaver's face, we had spent every day for the previous ten weeks in and out of her body. A clear plastic bag encircled her head, and a white muslin cloth, moistened with formaldehyde, clung to the contours that were her eyes, nose, and mouth. I lifted the cloth slowly, starting at the corner that covered her chin. Somehow I felt that seeing her face—her eyes, her lips, and her final expression—would confirm the life I had tried to re-create in my mind. Unlike her abdomen, our cadaver's face was smooth and the skin tight. Her chin appeared exquisitely chiseled, and her lips, still stained with a burnt-orange lipstick, were thin. Despite all the work we had done to the rest of her body over the previous two and a half months, our cadaver looked peaceful, asleep even.

Her eyes were closed. I lifted her right eyelid, wanting to know the color of her eyes, the windows through which she looked out into her world. The eyes, I hoped, would finally tell me the rest of her story. I would be able to look upon her as those who surrounded her during her life had. But there were no eyes under either her right or her left lid, just empty sockets. I had never seen enucleated bare sockets; and instead of being shocked, as I would have imagined, I felt a profound sadness, a kind of void, as if I had been robbed of closure to the imagined life of my cadaver. "She probably donated her corneas after death," said my professor.

Her eyes were not the only things that were taken away before her arrival to us. Her brain, the control center of her soul, had also been removed. "It's being saved for later," said our anatomy professor. "You'll dissect it next semester in neurology lab." The empty cranium, like the hollow eye sockets, looked like a room that had been hastily vacated.

We peeled away the skin on her face, uncovering the nerves and muscles that controlled the expressions she had used over a lifetime. I asked my lab partners to allow me to do this part of the dissection. Holding the small scalpel like a pencil, I separated and lifted the thin facial skin from the underlying muscles, a technique similar to that used in face-lifts. The dissection had to be done meticulously so as not to cut inadvertently any fine facial nerves or vessels. I found the work soothing; over the previous ten weeks I had come to enjoy this technical work of dissection, particularly the finer parts. Moreover, I wanted to spend more time with her face to see if I could piece together other parts of her life.

Unlike many of her other muscles, my cadaver's facial muscles turned out to be beautifully developed. I came to believe that she, even as she approached her death from ovarian cancer, embraced living; the strong muscles of her smile and around her eyes reflected someone who relished life's emotions. While the cancer had eaten away at the rest of her body, these muscles of facial expression survived and even flourished despite the hardships she surely faced.

Unbeknownst to me at that time, my cadaver, my very first patient, was much like my living patients that would follow. Pushed to view their own mortality directly, they too would live the remainder of their own lives that much more fully than the rest of us.

Our final anatomy exam came two weeks later. By this time, dissecting had long since become routine. We spent our free moments at night up in the labs with our cadavers, looking at parts and committing them to memory. If time was short, we ordered pizza after working for a couple of hours, ate quickly in the lab halls, then went back to dissect. The smell of formaldehyde had become a part of life, a badge of pride as we walked by other graduate students who recognized the smell and thus our place as students of medicine. For a brief moment during those twelve weeks we felt like true descendents of our medical forefathers, a part of the history of medicine that has remained unchanged for centuries. We were performing dissections similar to those that had been performed by Vesalius over four centuries before and documenting them within our brains. We came to believe that even in death, the human body contains the secrets of life. And like those great forefathers of medicine, we learned to suppress our instincts of fear and even of repulsion. We pushed those emotions out of our consciousness in order to further medical knowledge.

We had become initiated.

The afternoon after our final exam, I returned to the lab for one last visit with my cadaver. Laboratory technicians had spent the day preparing our cadavers for shipment, but the rooms were now quiet and empty. I opened the familiar latched door underneath the lab bench and pulled out the metal bed.

She was covered neatly in white plastic, ready to move to her final resting place. Through the plastic I touched her forehead, her shoulders, and her hands. I sat in my old jeans and high school T-shirt, thumbing through my memories of her body and the story it told us. I closed my eyes and envisioned her anatomy, referring to it as I would again innumerable times in my future practice. *Thank you,* I thought, feeling at that moment the strong and regular beats at the center of my own chest. *Thank you for your final gift.*

Intensive Care

DANIELLE OFRI

The patient was a routine alcoholic, hauled off the streets of Manhattan on a warm June evening and brought to the Bellevue emergency room. Or maybe he staggered into the ER. In either case, when his dose of Thunderbird or Mad Dog wore off, he slid into alcohol withdrawal. The ER staff probably gave him ten milligrams of Valium to stop the shakes and racing heart rate. Then twenty milligrams, then forty. Apparently they'd been unable to calm the tremors and agitation at even the highest doses of Valium, and so started giving him barbiturates—the "big guns." Eventually, they did silence his tremors and, in the process, his breathing. So by the time he arrived in our ICU, he was intubated with a breathing tube down his throat and a heaving ventilator at his side pushing in the oxygen. There was nothing else to do except wait out the days until the barbiturates wore off so we could extubate him and allow him to breathe on his own.

Now we stood in front of our patient in Bed 12, his disheveled street looks frozen in place by the barbiturate coma. Lauren was presenting the case. She was a shy, petite intern with a mousy demeanor. Dr. Sitkin, our lanky six-foot attending, slouched against the IV pole as she spoke, a derisive half-smile on his face the entire time. He shook his head slowly when she finally finished. "Jeez," he said, in his Tennessee drawl, "where do they unearth these ER docs? Haven't they ever read a textbook in their lives, or do they still use garlic cloves down there?" Lauren reddened and looked down quickly. "I'm serious now," Dr. Sitkin said, standing up and straightening out the slight hunch of his shoulders. "It's like hauling in a John Deere tractor to knock off a pesky moth. Now this guy ain't gonna be whistling Dixie for some time."

"What day is it today, anyway?" He glanced down at his watch. "June third? This guy ain't gonna wake up this week." His hands began to gesticulate in the air. "This guy ain't gonna wake up this month. This guy ain't gonna wake up until at least Rosh Hashana." He pointed to the ventilator. "In fact, why don't we just park a shofar on this ol' ventilator. When he starts blowing the shofar, we'll know it's time to extubate him."

I didn't want to do it. I didn't want to laugh in front of a patient. I didn't want to laugh *at* a patient. Again. But the image of our homeless alcoholic blowing the ram's horn in Bed 12 of the ICU just rocked my funny bone and, to my embarrassment and annoyance, I once again found myself laughing uncontrollably on rounds with Dr. Sitkin. I thought his humor was off-color, inappropriate, and sometimes downright insulting to the patients or the staff. But the combination of his dry Jewish humor and his Southern drawl just overpowered my self-control. In between his jokes, he freely peppered us with educational pearls. His breadth of knowledge extended way beyond his field of infectious diseases—he was always impressing us with arcane fungi and protozoa—to all of general internal medicine and critical care medicine. But he was equally free with his biting criticism for anyone who wasn't as smart or fast as he, which was most of the world.

Dr. Sitkin looked around at our team, which was a healthy mix of ethnicities and colors. His lean face screwed up in a smirk and his bushel of wiry salt-and-pepper hair cascaded over his brow. He eased his tiny wire-rimmed glasses low down on his bony nose and his eyes darted over the tops. "For the goyim amongst us, there's a copy of the Talmud in my office next to my other bible, Mandell's *Infectious Disease*. You can consult either one if you need a refresher on Rosh Hashana ritual." He shoved his glasses back up and sauntered on to the next patient.

"This one's dead," he said passing by my patient with metastatic esophageal cancer in Bed 11. "What's he doing in our ICU?"

"His daughter hasn't signed the DNR yet," I said.

"Rubbish. There's no rule about having to administer critical care to a corpse just because there's no DNR in place. You don't have to give medical care that's not warranted. Ship this guy out." On Dr. Sitkin marched, and our team jogged to catch up with his long strides.

"Dead. Dead. Dead," he pronounced, moving swiftly past the Alzheimer's patient with three strokes in Bed 10, the woman with metastatic lung cancer in Bed 9, and the demented bilateral amputee with renal failure and liver failure in Bed 8. On the days when our other attending, Dr. Marks, rounded with us, we spent a full ten minutes at each bedside reviewing the labs, the X-rays, and the medications. The poor prognosis would be acknowledged in an oblique way, but the entire treatment plan would be discussed and debated as with any other patient. Only Dr. Sitkin had the

honesty—or the chutzpah, depending on your viewpoint—
to call it like it was. "Dead. Dead. Dead. Why are we wasting our time even talking?" The team would shuffle along
uncomfortably, knowing that he was right in a way—all
these patients were going to die in the near future no matter
what we did—but it didn't seem proper, somehow, to say
that right out in the open.

Bed 11—"Dead." Bed 10—"Dead." Bed 9—"Dead."
Bed 8—"Dead." Bed 7. This was where Dr. Sitkin would
stop. Stop walking and stop joking. Li-Feng Chen was
thirty-two years old. Her leukemia had been in remission
for two years, but six months into her pregnancy it flared up
with a "blast crisis." Determined to keep her baby, she
avoided chemotherapy until she was so sick that she required
an emergency Caesarean section. The baby was downstairs
in the neonatal ICU; Ms. Chen was upstairs in the adult
ICU. Her bone marrow had been devastated by the leukemia and her body was now a veritable petri dish for
infection.

"This is a patient who deserves our ICU," Dr. Sitkin said.
"This is a patient who might be able to benefit from our
intensive monitoring." On the days we rounded with Dr.
Sitkin, we spent 98 percent of our time in front of Ms.
Chen's bed. He demanded to know every lab value, the
exact dose of every medication, the specific chemotherapy
regimen. He'd perch on the edge of the chart rack and grill
us on the minutiae of her care. And then he'd scrunch up his
face and think. Minutes of silence would follow as the whole
team watched him cogitate. He'd rub his nonexistent beard
or twirl the wedding ring around his finger. Then he'd say,
"I'm not satisfied with her antibiotic coverage. She's at risk
both from typical infections seen in oncology patients as
well as those from a gynecological source. Let's start from

scratch." He'd have us draw more blood cultures, repeat a spinal tap, change all of her IV lines, and then start her on new antibiotics.

On the railing of Ms. Chen's bed was a Polaroid picture of her baby. It was a scrawny thing with a full head of wet black hair, sporting nearly as many tubes and catheters as her mother. As we left Bed 7, I always thought I caught Dr. Sitkin stealing a glance at that photo.

Dr. Sitkin was not shy about sharing with us the latest exploits of Andrea, his eight-month-old. "Yesterday, she discovered her toes," he announced during a conference. "Don't ask me how she did it, but she managed to get all five of her toes in her mouth at once. The kid's a genius. My wife and I attempted the same thing, and I warn you . . . don't try this at home without the proper safety mechanisms."

One day, I had to choose which antibiotics to give to my patient with metastatic esophageal cancer after he had spiked a new fever. I debated which combination of drugs I should use, and then I thought, Gee, we have a specialist in infectious diseases this month, let me give him a call. I left a message at Dr. Sitkin's private-practice office, and he called back promptly. I described the situation and asked his advice.

"My advice is that you grow up and make your own decisions. Don't page me to choose some designer assortment of antibiotics. I don't care which ones you use, the patient's dead anyway." He hung up the phone and I felt ashamed of my juvenile question.

Every Wednesday, we had "ICU Touchy-Feely Rounds." One of the psychiatrists met with the residents over a pizza lunch to discuss any feelings we had about our time in the ICU. Our attendings were deliberately not present, so we could feel free to talk. Frequently, we bitched about the long hours.

Occasionally, someone talked about a difficult patient. But mostly we complained about Dr. Sitkin. About how inappropriate he could be. About his constant jokes at the expense of patients. About how we were made to be "colluders" in his humor. About how he had no patience for 95 percent of the staff and 95 percent of the patients. About how we were nervous presenting cases in front of him because he always had cutting criticism to offer.

On Wednesday afternoons, he'd catch my eye with a wink and say, "Did you all have a good time kvetching about me?" I would smile sheepishly, and he'd say, "That's okay. All of your complaints are probably justified—I'm a boor, I'm insensitive, I'm condescending."

I'd nod cautiously. "Well, a few things like that were mentioned."

"Good, good," he'd smile. "It's heartening to know that I'm not losing my touch."

I decided to take some risk and push a little bit. "Well, some people feel a little uncomfortable with all the jokes, Dr. Sitkin."

"Jokes? Every goddamn person here is dying. What else can you do but joke? You guys take everything so seriously. Relax a little."

"Some people are a little uncomfortable during the case presentations because you can come down so hard on them."

He shook his head in disbelief. "Listen, I'm never going to lie to anyone. You can trust me on that. Whaddya guys want, a goddamn kindergarten ice-cream party?"

I shrugged. "That wouldn't be so bad."

The next day, during conference, Dr. Sitkin hauled in twelve pints of Ben & Jerry's ice cream. "Ofri thinks I'm being too harsh on you," he announced, plunking them on the table one by one, their lids glistening with frost. "She thinks I should get you some ice cream to make you feel better." The room was silent for a moment. But residents are residents, and free food is free food, even if it was ice cream for breakfast. Everyone dove in with plastic spoons, competing for the good flavors like Chocolate Chip Cookie Dough and Super Fudge Chunk.

Dr. Sitkin licked a spoonful of vanilla. "How am I doing, Ofri?" he asked dryly. "Better?"

During our case conference the following week, Lauren was presenting one of the admissions from the previous night. Lauren could have passed for twelve years old. Everything about her—her wispy voice, her four-foot-ten height, her shyness, her wide, innocent eyes—appeared childlike. Dr. Sitkin's raucous sarcasm made her visibly nervous. Even though she'd grown up on the same side of the Mason-Dixon Line as he, she'd inherited the more genteel aspects of Southernism, while Dr. Sitkin was more of a Brooklynite cloaked in a Tennessee drawl.

Lauren read from her admission note. The note was long and overly detailed. Lauren's nervousness kept her from even once looking up from the printed page. She labored over word after word, too tense to include any inflection or pause. Even I couldn't deny that it was boring as she plodded along. We all were feeling the somnolent effects of her dry presentation, and struggled to stay focused. Dr. Sitkin rolled his eyes. Then he rolled his neck, loudly cracking a joint. Then he plunked his head on the table and left it there, curled up in his arms.

We sat in stunned silence. Slowly, we looked from one to the other. We'd never seen an attending do that before; nobody knew what to do. Lauren resumed reading from her admission note in a tentative voice, but Dr. Sitkin didn't stir.

Eventually her voice petered out and we sat riveted to our seats.

No one said or did anything to break the silence. Finally I took a deep breath. "Should we call a code?" I asked.

Smiles bubbled up on people's faces, but no one wanted to laugh out loud. Dr. Sitkin snapped his head upward and the team giggled, then burst out laughing. He looked at me, and I wasn't sure if it was a look of anger or humor. He nodded slowly. "Good one, Ofri. Touché."

Ms. Chen grew sicker. Her leukemia had spun out of control, taking her immune system with it; the infections were getting the best of her. Every morning on rounds, we sped through the ICU until Dr. Sitkin parked us at Bed 7. We ploughed through the data exhaustively, hunting for a chink in the relentless progression of her pathology through which we could intervene. "Leukemia can be a curable disease," Dr. Sitkin insisted. "If we can pull her through this crisis, she still might achieve a remission, if not a permanent cure. Forget all the corpses in the other beds; this is where our attention should be."

The nurses from the neonatal ICU paid visits frequently to update Ms. Chen on her daughter's condition. Ms. Chen had not seen her daughter since the birth, four weeks ago. She'd had a few minutes to meet her baby in the delivery room before each was whisked to her respective ICU. The Polaroids on the railing were updated weekly.

When Ms. Chen began to bleed from her gut, we transfused her. When she began to have seizures, we hauled her and all of her machinery downstairs for a head CT. When her lungs weakened, we intubated her and gave her a breathing tube.

"I only give up when there's no hope," Dr. Sitkin said. "And there's still hope." He still made "whale blubber" remarks about the obese demented lady in Bed 2. He still had no patience for the end-stage AIDS patient in Bed 3, even though a large portion of his private practice consisted of AIDS patients. "I have nothing against dying—it's a noble process—but it should be done at home or in a regular medical bed. Not in the ICU. This is the place to give intensive care when there is a possibility of meaningful recovery. We're not a hospice here."

On that Tuesday morning, when we told him that Ms. Chen had died overnight, Dr. Sitkin was quiet and only nodded. He asked us to tell him in detail what had happened. We described the incessant hemorrhaging and intractable fevers. We described the bottoming blood pressure that refused to respond to any intervention. We told him how her lungs flooded despite the forced air of the ventilator. We told him that her seizures continued unabated. We told him how we pronounced her dead at 4:53 a.m. and then called her family. He nodded throughout. "Good job," he said at the end, his voice uncharacteristically soft. "You guys did a good job."

On the last day of our month in the ICU, we sat with Dr. Sitkin in the conference room. "Okay, guys, here's your chance to tell me what you think of me. We're going around the room in ascending order of seniority—interns first. Be brutally honest, because that's how I'd be with you. And don't worry—anything you say today has probably been said before about me."

He pointed to Lauren. "You first."

Lauren immediately reddened.

"C'mon, Lauren. Lay it on the line. I ain't made of glass," he drawled.

Lauren cleared her throat. "Well, I appreciated all the stuff you taught us about infectious disease."

"Don't worry, you don't have to make me feel good."

"Well, sometimes you made me feel shy. You made me feel like I couldn't do anything good."

Dr. Sitkin nodded and twirled his wedding ring. "Good, good, now we're getting somewhere. Keep it coming."

"But I can do things good," she said.

"Tell me, Lauren. What can you do good?"

She paused. "I can sing."

"Sing?"

"Yes, I sing every Sunday in church."

Dr. Sitkin smiled and leaned back in his chair. "By all means, Lauren. Sing us a song."

Lauren looked at him, confused.

"I'm serious," Dr. Sitkin said. "Sing us a song."

Lauren adjusted her lab coat, then stood up slowly. She focused on a spot over our heads and opened her mouth. Out came the loudest, clearest soprano that I'd ever heard. All of her diffidence and "childlikeness" suddenly melted away. It was as though when she stood up those robes slipped away onto the chair behind her. She belted out a church hymn that was almost too powerful for our little conference room. We were jolted awake and mesmerized by this stunning, compelling woman before us. When she finished, she sat down abruptly.

Dr. Sitkin was visibly moved. "Thank you, Lauren. I'll have to say that's never happened to me before." Back in her seat, Lauren was as physically diminutive as she'd always been, but she never again appeared childlike to me.

Dr. Sitkin went around the room, pointing at each intern and then each resident, who gave him some feedback. When he got to me, he went out of order and skipped to the pulmonary fellow who was actually above me in seniority. "You're last, Ofri. I'm saving the best for last."

When it was finally my turn, the room quieted. Everyone seemed to expect a face-off, because they knew I had criticized him heavily both in person and in "Touchy-Feely Rounds."

"Well, Sitkin," I said. "This month has been nothing if not interesting. You have been a unique attending in all my time at Bellevue. I appreciate your honesty and I know that you really do care about the patients and us, even if you won't always admit to it." I took a deep breath. "But at times you are entirely inappropriate, juvenile, insulting, and downright nasty. I sometimes can't believe that the department lets you run free like this, entrusting the education of impressionable young interns to you. And I hate the way you make fun of sick patients who are dying. I think that's despicable."

"Whew," Dr. Sitkin said. "I was worried for a moment that you were actually going to say something bad about me."

"The worst thing is," I continued, "is that I find your disgusting humor incredibly funny and I've actually enjoyed this month in the ICU."

"Praise the Lord," he said, looking upward. "She likes me. Ofri actually likes me."

I had been visiting a friend at the beach on Long Island one weekend in early August, and biked over to the Amagansett Farmers Market to pick up some bagels. Sitting on one of the wooden benches by a bin of freshly harvested corn were Dr. Sitkin and his wife. A racing bike leaned against the back of the bench. When he saw me, he smiled and beckoned me over.

"Julie," he said to his wife, "this is Danielle Ofri, one of the best residents from Bellevue."

A compliment from Sitkin? An honest-to-goodness compliment? It took me a moment to absorb what he'd just said, and then I could feel a goofy grin spread from ear to ear, but I couldn't help it. A compliment from Sitkin. When I recovered from my shock, I reached out and shook hands with his wife. "It's a pleasure to meet you. Your husband is a one-of-a-kind attending."

Julie smiled. "He certainly is a one-of-a-kind guy. And you must be a one-of-a-kind resident if you managed to survive with him and still come out smiling."

"We actually had a lot of fun in the ICU," I said. "Do you come out here often?"

"We have a house here, in East Hampton," Julie said. "Most weekends we're here, though, Joseph spends more time on his bike than in the house."

"That's not true," Dr. Sitkin said in mock protest. "Just once a day, I take a spin to Sag Harbor to stretch my legs." East Hampton to Sag Harbor was twenty miles round-trip, and it wasn't all flat.

"Hey, Ofri," Dr. Sitkin said, "you haven't met the most important members of the family." He lifted a baby out of the stroller that was parked next to the bench. "This little sweetheart is Andrea." He cradled her in his arms and tickled her chin so she would smile at me.

"Ah, yes, the one who can get all her toes in her mouth."

"Precisely. And the real genius of the family is Ellen. Ellen? Where are you hiding?"

A doe-eyed four-year-old came bounding out of the

nearby wooden dollhouse and leaped onto the bench next to
him. "This is Ellen," Dr. Sitkin said. "She's going to be a
nephrologist when she grows up."

"I like kidneys," Ellen announced.

"I like kidneys, too," I said, "and it's a pleasure to meet
you."

We chatted for ten minutes about my upcoming board
exams, the new deck they were building on their home, and
the receding dunes on the beach. When I'd finished my coffee, I bid them goodbye and hopped on my bike. I didn't
often have a chance to socialize with my attendings. It felt
nice. It felt like I was actually growing up.

Eighteen months later, I was returning home from a two-
week vacation in Israel. It was a chilly January morning,
and I was walking down Broadway on the Upper West Side.
I had arrived only yesterday and I was still jet-lagged, but
not jet-lagged enough to pass up a quarter-pound of Zabar's
best lox. My mind was tired, and it wandered from the British Airways billboard to the posters advertising upcoming
rock concerts at Madison Square Garden. I saw a Missing
Person flyer posted on a streetlamp for a young college student who had disappeared from a New Year's Eve party.
Probably overdosed on drugs, I thought, and walked past it.
Then the thought suddenly struck me—that flyer represented a person. And not only a person, it represented a
family in emotional panic. That kid was somebody's son,
somebody's baby. How could I just walk by? A block away
was another lamppost with another flyer posted on it, and I
walked deliberately over to it. I was going to pay these poor
souls their due. The white photocopied paper was affixed
with tape on the top and bottom, but the corners flew loose

in the wind. Suddenly I found myself staring at the face of Joseph Sitkin. "Missing," it said, "since Monday. Last seen wearing blue jeans and yellow parka." The photo showed his trademark curly hair spilling over the edges of his wire-rimmed glasses.

I felt my legs grow weak as I grabbed the lamppost for support. I was sure my vision had been mistaken. These Missing Person flyers were always filled with distorted photos of strangers whose presence or absence could not affect my life. There must have been some mistake.

I pulled myself back up and forced my eyes to gaze upon the flyer again. The photocopied version of the picture blurred the details and one couldn't make out the sharp wit and ample intelligence that I knew permeated the lean features of his face, but it was Dr. Sitkin, or at least a representation of Dr. Sitkin. It was a disembodied reflection of the man I knew, not just because of the warped physical details of the picture, but because of his very presence on such a poster. I felt like I was looking through a photographic negative, and there was something discomfortingly unbalanced about seeing the opposite of presence. I was staring at his absence. How could Dr. Sitkin be missing?

I spotted an acquaintance on the street, someone not in the medical field, and I pointed out the flyer, asking if she had heard about this. "Oh, yes," she said. "It's been all over the news this week. His wife was on TV and everything."

How could I have been so out of touch with the news while I was in Israel?

I raced to the medical school library where I knew that a week's worth of the *New York Times* would remain stashed on a shelf before being discarded. I flipped furiously through the pages of the back issues until I stumbled upon the headline "Prominent Manhattan Doctor Missing from Upper

West Side Apartment." I scanned the text desperately. "Dr. Joseph Sitkin was last seen Monday morning." "Always jogged in the early mornings." "Nothing missing from apartment." "No sign of foul play."

In the issue two days later there was another article, entitled "Missing Doctor Left Note on Computer." My heart pounded as I read on. "The letter on Dr. Sitkin's computer spoke of his despondency." Despondency? The man who always had a joke on hand? The man who marveled at his daughter's ability to fit all of her toes in her mouth? "Dr. Sitkin's long, rambling letter chronicled his increasing despair as well as his love for his wife and two daughters."

The newspapers crumpled in my hand and I crumpled in my seat. How could this have happened? Were there any signs? Could we have known? Or helped? For the next week, there was a palpable tension at the medical center. Rumors circulated that Dr. Sitkin had had a nervous breakdown and was recuperating somewhere anonymously. Someone said there was a report of a credit card purchase in East Hampton and that he must be out at their summer home.

On January 29, two weeks from the date of his disappearance, a body washed ashore. "A badly decomposed body was found on the rocks," the *New York Times* read the next day, "under the Manhattan side of the George Washington Bridge yesterday, and the police tentatively identified it as that of Dr. Joseph Sitkin, a prominent Manhattan doctor who disappeared two weeks ago and left a note—"

I closed my eyes from the headlines, unable to read on. How could it have felt, I agonized to myself, to stand on that bridge in the early chill of the morning and stare down at the Hudson River swirling below? How much must his heart have ached as his palm rested upon the frigid metal handrail? With how much despair must his legs have trembled as he eased his athletic limbs over the edge? How much anguish must he have possessed to combat the vertiginous assault of facing down the furious river?

I could only put my hand over my mouth and clamp my already closed eyes even further shut to block out the vision of his final moments. But I couldn't erase the internal vision of his pain and that of his wife, Julie. I shuddered at the thought of that icy moment of transition from her annoyance at his being late to her panic at his absence. The distraught days of unknowing, like a slowly cranked torture rack. The discovery of his letter, of the worst fears confirmed. And the baffling illogic of the world to render this comprehensible to two little girls.

The next day I found myself crammed in the downtown No. 1 train with the press of morning commuters. I slithered open my *New York Times* just a crack to peek at the news. I found myself at the obituaries, and there it was: "Sitkin, Joseph, beloved husband of Julie, devoted father of Andrea and Ellen, dead at the age of 39. According to his wishes, the family has donated his body to the Microbiology Department at NYU Medical Center." It was suddenly so real, so final. I began to sniffle and swallow. And then the tears began to creep out. Someone offered me a seat and suddenly I began to cry unabashedly. The commuters looked on in helpless confusion. A woman asked me if I was feeling okay. I pointed to the obituary and said, "I knew him. That doctor from NYU who's been missing, I knew him. He was one of my teachers." And I bawled openly amidst the embarrassed silence of the subway car.

I escaped from the subway and walked the remaining thirty blocks home. Thirty painful blocks. Thirty blocks of remembering the comatose alcoholic with the shofar by his side and the twelve pints of Ben & Jerry's ice cream for breakfast. Thirty blocks of remembering how Dr. Sitkin encouraged Lauren's powerful song, and the way he always glanced at the Polaroid photo of Ms. Chen's baby, taped to the railing of Bed 7. Thirty blocks of remembering how he made me laugh and how I actively struggled to dislike him and just couldn't. Thirty blocks of remembering the tough work and the extraordinary payoff of earning Dr. Sitkin's respect.

Ours is a dangerous profession, I've often thought. There is the constant assault of physical and emotional challenges of taking care of patients, which is layered upon the already difficult task of conducting our own lives. It is no wonder that so many of us become overwhelmed at times and need some intensive care. For every Dr. Sitkin who eventually declares his pain to the world, there are probably fifty others who suffer silently, for whom the anguish burns slowly and excruciatingly. The medical profession has little room or patience for hearing about this. These feelings often get expressed as bitter, abusive personalities, or drug and alcohol addictions.

The cliché says that doctors make the worst patients, that they are the last to seek treatment. We are always trying to help our patients get beyond their denial, but it seems that we use it the most for ourselves. Is that the Faustian bargain we make when we enter the profession? I don't want to believe that is true, but for some it is apparently so.

Falling Down

SANDEEP JAUHAR

On call nights, the ward was like a sleeping village, and you were the night watchman on patrol with your penlight and stethoscope. Senior residents were available for backup, but after 10:00 p.m. they were almost always admitting patients or at home sleeping. You could call them if you needed help, but few of us ever did. Not calling backup, I quickly learned, was considered a sign of strength, and for an intern there was nothing more flattering than to be considered "strong." Once, I made the mistake of calling a third-year resident at her apartment in the middle of the night to ask for help performing a spinal tap. She roared at me on the phone for not taking care of the procedure earlier, before she came on duty at 10:00 p.m. When she arrived on the floor, she quickly saw my patient, told me a tap was unnecessary, and then berated me some more for wasting her time. I never called another resident for the remainder of the year, paging Rajiv instead (in the middle of the night, if necessary) when I needed help. If I could get so much flak asking for help managing a potential case of meningitis, I could only imagine the kind of wrath I'd incur calling about atypical chest pain or something equally benign.

On night duty, it wasn't the emergencies that overwhelmed so much as the little things, the minor issues—the insomnia, the constipation, the headaches—that the nurses had to make you aware of in the middle of the night. Even when the nurses didn't call, it was impossible to enter any sort of restful sleep. The expectation of the pager going off was enough to keep you in a state of chronic anxiety. Sometimes I'd pace back and forth in the call room, or just outside in the corridor, looking out the window onto the East River and the points of yellow light dotting the skyscape, wondering what sort of calamity would next be visited on me. If I did fall asleep, I usually woke up with a drenching wetness on the back of my neck. Once, a nurse called to tell me that a young man, nervous about a procedure scheduled for the morning, had had fleeting chest pain. When I saw him, he was visibly nervous but otherwise fine. When I told the nurse that a twinge of chest discomfort in an otherwise healthy young man did not require an *extensive* workup, she made it clear that if I didn't at least perform an electrocardiogram, she was going to file a complaint. So I went and got a machine and wheeled it to the patient's room, but it was broken, and I went and got another one on a different ward, but it was broken, too, and by the time I performed the EKG forty-five minutes later, the patient was fast asleep and irritated at being woken and, of course, his EKG was completely normal.

There were set times on call when you could expect a flurry of pages, like when the nurses checked vital signs at 4:00 a.m. That was when they called about fevers. Your response was always the same: blood and urine cultures and a portable chest X-ray to rule out pneumonia. But sometimes you discovered that a patient was already on antibiotics or that blood cultures had been drawn every night for the past week, every single one negative, and then you had to decide whether you really needed to stick him again, but most of the time you did so anyway, not for the patient's sake but for your own, lest someone fault you in the morning for not doing it. That was the sad reality of residency: much of the time you were ordering tests to protect yourself. "The endgame of life is so depressing," I wrote in my diary. "Look at Mr. Fisher. Successful lawyer, Goldberg patient. Now look at him. Sick, febrile, dying of who-knows-what: cancer, TB, sarcoidosis? If you think about it, it could make all of life seem unworthwhile if, in the end, we end up dying in the hospital, awakened at 4:00 a.m. by a stupid intern trying to draw another set of blood cultures."

Sometimes I worried about how I was going to get through another night on call, until I realized that my patients were helping me. Their bodies had homeostatic reserve, the capacity to self-correct, to compensate for my mistakes. In physics, an oscillator quickly returns to its equilibrium position after being displaced, and so it is, I came to believe, with the human body. Most of my patients were going to be fine despite anything I did, and if they were going to die—well, that was probably going to happen despite me, too. Health was like the wilderness: it could only be spoiled by human intervention. "We're not saving patients," Rajiv told me. "We're just stabilizing them so they can save themselves."

I became awed by this concept, but most of my colleagues seemed indifferent to it. We performed our interventions with such confidence, such arrogance, but most of the time there was no way of predicting whether we were doing the right thing, or even a good thing. We'd give potassium for hypokalemia, or diuretics for edema, or nitroglycerin for high blood pressure—and we would overshoot. The diuretics would make our patients dehydrated or the nitroglycerin would lower their blood pressure too much—and then we'd have to give them intravenous fluid or raise their blood pressure with other drugs, and the process would start all over again. Sometimes we would give drugs just to treat the side effects of other drugs. Sometimes we would do illogical things like giving fluid and diuretics at the same time, and no one questioned it, including me. There was too much going on, too much complexity, to start asking questions. I wasn't sure where to begin; I wasn't even sure I knew enough to know what to ask. My energy was low, my enthusiasm flagging, and the system was in automatic drive anyway. The easiest thing to do was to get out of the way.

When the nurses woke you in the middle of the night, you had to be prepared to deal with the unexpected. You knew that energy, clarity, fluent speech were coming; you just didn't know when. One night, I was half asleep when I got paged. *Must be blood culture time,* I thought, reaching for the phone. In the dark, the receiver vibrated like an image from a jittery screen projector. When I called the number on my beeper, an urgent voice told me to go to Mrs. MacDougal's room. When I got there, it was as if I had walked in on a play. Mrs. MacDougal was standing precariously in the middle of her private room in a puddle of urine. Bright ceiling lights were beating down on her like stage spotlights. She was an attractive woman, for ninety-one, with a sharp patrician nose and handsome cheekbones like Lauren Bacall's. Her gown was open in the back, exposing her scoliotic torso, which was covered with age spots, like cow patties in a field. A nurse and two orderlies were circling her like muggers. They were trying to get her to go back to bed, but the old woman was insisting on going to the bathroom alone.

"We'll help you go in the bedpan," someone said, grabbing her arm to keep her from falling.

"I want to go to the bathroom!" she shrieked, trying to wriggle free.

"We can't let you walk there."

"I'm not going in the bed!"

"You're going to slip and fall."

"Leave me be!"

I was trying to keep from falling over myself. I tried reasoning with Mrs. MacDougal, but she wouldn't listen to me, either. After a couple of minutes of urging, I asked the nurse why we couldn't just let her go to the bathroom.

"She could break her hip," the nurse said indignantly.

"She could, but I don't think she will," I replied.

"I can go by myself!" Mrs. MacDougal cried.

"I know," I said, "but let me walk you anyway." I offered her the crook of my arm and, much to my amazement, this appeal to her ladylike instincts seemed to work. Off we went, with an aide on either side, to the toilet.

An aide went in with her while the rest of us waited outside. "She's sundowning," the nurse said, clearly irritated, referring to a kind of nocturnal delirium often observed in nursing homes. "Before you leave, order restraints."

"Do you think that's necessary?" I asked skeptically.

"What if she sundowns again?"

"Just call me," I replied. People in the hospital were always obsessing about disasters that never occurred. I had seen it myself in the CCU, where nurses would use PRN ("as-needed") sedative orders to keep patients groggy and cooperative through the night.

When Mrs. MacDougal came out, I walked her back to bed. "You're a nice young man," she said.

"Thank you," I replied.

"I like you."

"Well, I like you, too." That was the nicest thing I had

heard all week. I was going to show these nurses that a little kindness could go a long way. The next page came about forty-five minutes later. When I arrived back in the room, the scene was much the same as before, except now Mrs. MacDougal was standing in a slurry of feces. She was yelling some of the vilest obscenities—"Cocksuckers! Mother-fuckers!"—that I had ever heard from a nonagenarian's lips. The stench was overpowering. I cupped my hand over my face, but the putrid odor still registered in my olfactory lobes.

"Mrs. MacDougal!" I cried through my fingers. "What are you doing?"

"Who the hell are you?" she screamed hoarsely.

"Dr. Jauhar!" I said, incredulous. "Don't you remember me? You promised you were going to stay in bed."

"I need to go to the bathroom."

I ordered her back to bed immediately.

"You're not my doctor!" she shouted. "Call Silverman. Tell him to get me out of here."

I told her that Dr. Silverman wasn't available.

"Get out of my way," she cried, swinging wildly at me. She slipped and fell into my arms, rubbing brown excrement onto my scrubs. Steadying myself, I felt my right sandal slide a bit. The nurses were looking at me with I-told-you-so satisfaction.

For a moment, I fantasized about putting Mrs. MacDougal into a choke hold and dragging her by the neck to bed, elbowing the nurse and orderlies out of the way, hissing, screaming at them to end this godforsaken shitfest. But, of course, that couldn't happen; I had to deal with the situation calmly. "Give her five of Haldol and two of Ativan," I shouted out as I tried to keep her from tipping over.

"Yes, Doctor," the nurse responded sarcastically before

going out to get the medicine. The two aides and I managed to force her back to bed. When the nurse returned, she administered two intramuscular injections. Almost immediately, Mrs. MacDougal stopped struggling. Within minutes, she was snoring heavily. I felt momentary relief, until the reading from the pulse oximeter started to drop: 99 . . . 98 . . . 97 . . . Pretty soon an oxygen mask was plastered to her face and I was turning a knob counterclockwise on the wall. 94 . . . 93 . . . 92 . . . The brief calm quickly turned into another round of panic. Why had I been so impulsive? Was there an antidote for Haldol? Should I call an ICU consult? Where were the nurses now? For the next couple of hours I remained at her bedside, watching her snort like a pig. I stabbed her wrist with a needle to get an arterial blood gas, which revealed borderline oxygen and carbon dioxide levels. I prayed the drugs would wear off. Why had I allowed myself to be goaded so rashly? In an effort to protect her (or perhaps myself), I was afraid that I had killed her. It was an apt metaphor for my internship thus far.

By the next morning, Mrs. MacDougal had returned to her sweet, great-grandmotherly self. At lunchtime a few days later, nurses, social workers, and people with nondescript titles like "coordinating manager" met to discuss patient "disposition"—who was going to be able to go home, who was going to require long-term care, and so on. Rohit told me to attend on his behalf. At the meeting, everyone seemed to be having a rollicking good time talking about the patients, exchanging gossip about family dynamics, and so on. The subject of Mrs. MacDougal came up. "Dr. Jauhar had a wrestling match with her a few nights ago," a social worker said, and everyone laughed except me. Someone asked where Mrs. MacDougal was going to go once she left the hospital. Her daughter wanted to put her in a nursing home, but she wanted to go back to living independently. "No way that's going to happen," someone said with a certitude I found troubling. Someone asked me for my opinion. I had had so little interaction with her, just one unfortunate incident, that I wasn't sure how to respond. I was wary of saying anything that could send her to a nursing home for the rest of her life. She had been delirious, no doubt, and a danger to herself, but she had also been in an unfamiliar environment with people she thought were trying to hurt her. Surely that had to enter the calculus for predicting future behavior. It was anyone's guess what she would be like in a more familiar environment. Wouldn't putting her into an institution just increase the likelihood of further sundowning? I thought of the Chekhov story "Ward No. 6," and the incarceration of Yefimitch. I did not want to be responsible for institutionalizing another person. I had seen it before on the psychiatry wards. If someone said they were well enough to go home, we would say they lacked insight into their disease and keep them even longer. Where was Dr. Silverman? I wondered. We were discussing the future of a stranger over sandwiches and soft drinks. And that was beginning to seem normal.

Beauty

GABRIEL WESTON

From my earliest days at medical school, I found surgery not just practical but beautiful. Dating from that first operation, when I had seen my tutor's brother replacing a cranky hip joint with a new one, this sense of surgery's fine aesthetic gathered momentum during the early years of my clinical education. Compared to the limitlessly difficult and ambiguous world of medicine, surgery was diagnostically clear. Relatively few surgical diseases were described, all of them concerned with quite definite abnormalities. Tumors, fractures, clots. Empirically true, often touchable facts.

The operations designed to treat these frailties were also lovely in their combination of regularity with a magical kind of artistry. In surgical textbooks, I found difficult procedures dissected and laid out in stages. They suggested a craft which was repeatable, reliable, and always dramatic. This last fact mattered to me. Being a surgeon just sounded so much more impressive than being a physician.

But the feature of surgery that struck me as most beautiful was its almost-military adherence to the principle of order. Surgeons started their days an hour earlier than their medical counterparts, and did ward rounds quickly and efficiently. Diseases were easy to diagnose, leaving time for the careful planning of classic procedures, tweaked to suit the individual patient. These operations were then performed with marvelous precision. Cure was not guaranteed, but decisive surgery was often a person's best chance of reaching that goal.

I observed the objective correlative of this philosophy in the immaculate layout of the operating theater. The geography was of a main room with annexes. Most important of these was the anesthetic room, where the patient goes to be put to sleep so as to avoid the stress of seeing where he or she is going to be cut open. The prep room is another ante-chamber, where the scrub nurse sorts through the pack of instruments, each operation with its own pack, with its own designated tools. Then there is the alcove for scrubbing, with its zinc sink and shelves piled with plastic-packed gowns and gloves in all sizes, in waxy paper envelopes.

I had enjoyed watching the choreography that animated this space many times. The way the anesthetic doors would open to deliver a bedded, tubed patient at the same time as the scrub nurse appeared with her trolley, like a hostess bringing out a science-fiction tea. And how the surgeon would enter center-stage, arms held aloft, gown billowing like a gust-filled kite.

I suppose I was in love, seeing beauty all around me in my new surgical world. It would not take long for me to see that surgery was not always rosy, not always controllable and pretty.

I was due to spend the evening in Accident and Emer-gency (A&E), shadowing a senior house officer (SHO) on his night shift. As a mere student, I had no responsibility. I was there to learn what I could, and to assist the junior doc-tor I had been assigned to, in whatever way he saw fit. To get a feel for this environment that would soon be like home.

That evening I was with a junior doctor called John. He was a conventional tubby guy, but I remember how attractive he seemed to me. After all, he was a real doctor and, although I was due to become one within months, the chasm of experience and style seemed huge between us. It's funny how doctors go from being really sexy when you're not one yourself to rather unsexy when you are.

Well, he was busy and at a loss for what to do with me. So he suggested that I go and take a history and do an examination on a man he had just seen, who had come in with abdominal pain. As John was telling me what to do, he was busy organizing an intravenous urethrogram on the same patient, a scan which I knew was routinely performed on those thought to have a kidney stone. I felt disappointed that I already knew the diagnosis on the person I was about to see. What was the point in reading an Agatha Christie story if you already knew who the murderer was? I thought, as I headed for cubicle 5.

I paused just outside the cubicle curtain, to collect myself, and to check, in my *Oxford Handbook,* vade mecum of all medical students, what questions I needed to ask someone with abdominal discomfort. I saw the usual list of factors germane to any sort of pain: onset, site, severity, duration, intensity, character, relieving or exacerbating factors. Plus the relevance of bladder and bowel habit. Then, conscious of trying to look less awkward than I felt, I went in.

The couple I introduced myself to were Mr. Cooke and his wife. He was sitting on the bed, and she was sitting on the chair beside it. Despite being in his late sixties, he was trim. Sitting back at a 45-degree angle had not produced a little roll of fat at his belt line. His face was not the florid hue of the cardiopath; his measured breathing suggested good lungs. Only a double furrow on his brow indicated discomfort. That and the fact that his eyes were closed as if he was trying to narrow his sensory field. His hair was gray and thin, but looked windswept rather than straggly. He was wearing khaki trousers. Not genteel chinos, but made of something thicker and more practical, like canvas.

On his top half, he wore a plaid shirt whose sleeves were rolled to just above the elbow so that I could see slim but sinewy arms, finished with large, strong hands. His knuckles were like big marbles, and his veins looked like tree roots, as if they wouldn't be soft if you pressed them with a finger of childlike curiosity. He was a slight man, but valor vied with slightness to be noticed first.

Next to him, his wife appeared almost buxom. She had a good bosom, and it had that stiff, unified look that made it hard to imagine that it was composed of two soft breasts. She had brown hair that was only just beginning to gray. It reached her shoulders, and some of it was held from her roughened cheek with a clip, which might have looked absurdly girlish but didn't, because her eyes, which met mine the instant that I walked into the room, had a shiny sort of wisdom in them.

It was hard to see exactly what she was wearing, since the folds of this merged into the creases and swaths of that, but it was all dark and soft, in grays and greens and browns, so that she looked wholesome and foresty. She had a handbag by her feet which stood up by itself. One of the handles was upright, and the other had collapsed to one side. And on her lap she had one of those old mauve-and-white Penguins that they now design mugs from, and this one was Virginia Woolf's *A Room of One's Own*. Mrs. Cooke looked as if she had had such a room all her life, or as if she had never needed one.

Because she was looking at me, I introduced myself more to her than him. He had opened his eyes when I entered the cubicle, but had closed them again when he heard the words "medical student," although with a kind smile. I might have felt put out, but Mrs. Cooke, in the same measure that her husband had dismissed me, welcomed me with her response. She gave me the kind of look that a governess might give a child that has just washed its hands adequately, and she closed her book. She put her book in her bag and then sat up, hands in lap, to give me her full attention. Her hands, too, looked strong. The skin on them was chapped like a gardener's. I thought briefly of the minute, unfair discrepancy: that a man's strong hands are alluring, but that beautiful hands in a woman are those that have done nothing.

She was patient with my questions, but we both knew that a diagnosis had already been made, so the interview felt sluggish. I dreaded the prospect of having to examine this dignified man in front of his owl-like wife. I didn't like to think of touching, let alone hurting, the abdomen that lay under that soft shirt. An abdomen which, in my imagination, grew intensely white and private.

So I was grateful when, by some happy conversational torque, things turned from the medical matter in hand to a discussion of poetry. I cannot remember how this happened. It turned out that Mr. Cooke was a retired professor of English literature, and once we left the subject of his own cranky body behind to turn to what interested him most, he became quite animated. His wife explained that they were engaged in a marriage-long dispute about the comparative merits of Augustan versus Romantic poetry. It must have been a sort of harbor, for they began to banter lightly about it now, he sometimes opening his eyes to praise Keats or Shelley, or especially Wordsworth, over her favorites, the champion of whom appeared to be Alexander Pope.

Mrs. Cooke's face had softened, and she was saying, "Oh, for goodness sake, Charles, all those ghastly demonstrations of feeling. All that narcissism. How can you . . ."

And he was chuckling, despite his still-closed eyelids. He reached for his wife's hand and found it easily. Grasping it in midair, he gave it a sort of playful shake up and down while he addressed me with, "My wife loves Pope with all his strictures and his order. Because she finds the chaos of the really great poets a bit too scary."

I noticed their hands, which stayed within the joint grip they had made, for a few seconds after his last quip. Her scuffed red skin. His bony fingers. The difference between them. Then they had to let go because of the discomfort of his having to extend his arm off the bed with no support.

I was trying to think of a way I could join in their conversation when Mr. Cooke's face suddenly seemed to fold in on itself, and an exclamation of pain rang from him. There was sweat on his face where there hadn't been before, and he didn't look good. I got up, tripping slightly on my chair, and rushed to find John or a nurse.

Within two minutes, Mr. Cooke had been wheeled into Resus, his wife as near to him as she could get, given the sudden interest of all the doctors and nurses taking him there, expediting this short journey. The space was compassed in a matter of seconds. Then Mr. Cooke was being hooked up to all sorts of things, and people were saying how low his blood pressure was, how tachycardic his pulse was. Even in my student ignorance, I could tell he was in hemodynamic shock, he looked so gray and unwell.

A senior A&E doctor, realizing that the diagnosis of ureteric colic had been wrong, performed a quick abdominal ultrasound right there, and this showed that Mr. Cooke had a leaking abdominal aortic aneurysm. Unless he was taken immediately to have this most major of all blood vessels in the body repaired, he would not survive the next hour.

At that point, I noticed several things at once. A nurse, calling theater to prepare them. The sight of John in the background, looking as if he was about to cry. The A&E registrar telling me that they needed extra hands in the theater, that none of his juniors were available, and that I should go and help. The bang of the A&E doors as Mr. Cooke's bed was bashed through them to take him to the theater. The sight of his wife, still relegated to the outer circle of bodies, standing in Resus, as the bed and her husband disappeared down the corridor. Trying to compose herself. Waiting for someone to tell her what she should do, where she should go.

I took a shortcut to theater, and changed hurriedly. They need me! I thought as I grabbed a blue cap from the cardboard box on top of the lockers on my way out of the women's changing room. Because I was alone, I allowed myself to feel the great excitement of the surgery I was about to assist in. I knew the operation would be dramatic, but had no doubt it would work. I was glad to be a part of this drama, and felt good even to be wearing surgical scrubs, a sense of pride I confess I still have whenever I don this costume, even since it has become my habit. I slowed my step as I approached the emergency theater, so that I wouldn't look breathless and uncool when I got there.

What I saw when I walked into the room shocked me and made me feel ashamed of my recent excitement. There was a scrum of blue backs leaning over Mr. Cooke on the operating table. He was neither undressed nor asleep, but the men in blue were working on him. One was cutting his shirt off, and others were leaning on him, forcing him to lie down, despite his efforts to rise up and scram. I saw his slim, muscular belly, that part of him I had been reluctant to expose half an hour before, and I noticed the little red Campbell de Morgan spots on its skin, just like my dad has.

Two men took one arm each. Other helpers brought arm-rests, which were fixed to the side of the operating table with large screws. Then Mr. Cooke's arms were forced down at his sides, an immoral arm-wrestle, one man fighting two. Once overcome, his arms were strapped in position like you sometimes see in old films about madhouses.

And there was the most dreadful noise. Mr. Cooke, previously so self-contained, was roaring like a bear. Then, as he was defeated, loud man-sobbing. And then this patient, pinned down in a position that reminded me of the Crucifixion, was attacked again, from another angle. An anesthetist moved in unseen from north of his head, and his futile flailing started again as he felt the insult of a thick needle being pushed into one of his bulging neck veins. This was the central line, through which he would be monitored, as well as the conduit for receiving drugs and fluids.

At the same time, two surgeons were daubing his narrow front with brown Betadine in massive painty sweeps. Mr. Cooke's legs were kicking a bit and his eyes were rolling all around, their luminous whites blindly scanning the activities taking place upon his powerless body. I didn't know who either of the surgeons was; only that one was a consultant and one a registrar. They didn't know who I was, either, but I was asked to scrub and became one of two assistants. I was told where to stand, on the patient's right-hand side, next to the other helper. On the opposite side of the table were the vascular consultant and his registrar.

The operation began with the swiftest laparotomy incision I have ever seen, the very first I had witnessed at that early stage in my training. In one concerted movement, the consultant literally sliced Mr. Cooke open, from xiphister-num to pubis. His proficiency was marvelously apparent to me: his decisiveness, his knowledge of exactly how much pressure to apply to the large blade to penetrate skin and subcutaneous tissue, without harming any important under-lying structures.

With another single effort, the boss hoisted the whole gut out of Mr. Cooke's abdominal cavity and dumped it uncer-emoniously on my side of the table. This forced me, and the guy I was standing next to, to huddle together, to form a barricade with our two adjacent bodies, to stop the snaking mass of small and large bowel from slipping between us, or around either of us, onto the floor. Arms outspread, we held its writhing bulk, and I will never forget the eerie move-ments it made, vermiculating in our joint embrace.

Looking down, I peered into the trough of Mr. Cooke's emptied abdomen, and could see it filling with blood so fast that the outline of the gushing source was visible beneath the red meniscus. Like when you fill a paddling pool with a hose and it's half full, and you can see a knuckle shape on the surface just above where the hose is. I had been given two huge suctions, and was holding their broad snouts into the crimson depths, one in each hand. These pipes were doing such a strong job that I could feel the pull of them sucking at the blood, and I could hear no milkshake-slurping noise from them; they were not wasting time sucking up a cocktail of air with the fluid, they were just hungrily suck-ing blood.

For the next minute or so, nothing seemed to happen. The clearing of blood could not keep up with the rate at which more flowed from the leaking aorta. I was remember-ing, from my cadaveric dissection days, the first time I had seen this enormous vessel. It is as thick as a walking stick, and stands plumb in the center of the body. It even has the same handle-shaped curve as it leaves its origin in the heart. From there, it travels all the way through the chest and abdomen down to the pelvis, where it bifurcates into the leg-supplying iliac arteries. I knew from my recent studies how few previously undiagnosed leaking aortic aneurysms are survived.

As if abandoning hope that he was ever going to get a clear view, the consultant splashed in, holding a weighty instrument. When his hands resurfaced, they were empty, because he had used this instrument to clamp the aorta. Then he asked for the Dacron graft, a piece of tubing to replace the leaking bit of vessel. This looked like one of those concertina-type tubes that plumb washing machines. I was given a huge retractor to hold to keep the abdomen wide open, and I would remain like this for the next three hours.

During that time, repeated attempts to make the graft work failed. Each time the boss undid the clamp, to check the patency of the anastomosis, blood poured into the abdominal cavity again.

I confess that, when at four in the morning the consultant announced there was no more he could do, my main feeling was relief. The hours in theater had piled up against the thirty minutes or so I had spent with Mr. Cooke in A&E, so that my short connection with him felt out of date. So that any sense of sentiment I might have had had been eclipsed by the drama of the night. And even the drama now felt jaded. I was just tired, and my arms hurt from holding the retractor for so long.

No one had spoken to me during this theater episode; so, once we had all stepped back from our meddling, it was easy for me to leave quickly. I didn't want to see Mr. Cooke's blood brim over, or to hear it disrupt the silence of new death with its splish-splash on the floor.

After changing, and on my way out of the theater suite, I happened to pass the relatives' room. Through the window, inlaid within its wooden, school-style door, I could see the broad back of the vascular consultant, a trapezoid imprint of sweat on his scrub top. And then I heard the sudden, uncontrolled noise of Mrs. Cooke's first exhalation of grief, as horrible as the last sounds her husband had ever made, while struggling to resist the anesthetic. Unheard by him, as he had been by her. Standing outside the room, outside of that immediate extreme zone, I felt embarrassed by the noise before it saddened me. In the way that the sound of people having sex in a nearby hotel room might embarrass you before having any other effect.

Then I saw the top of Mrs. Cooke's head, mostly obscured from view by the consultant's shoulder. She had got up, and she must have been hitting his chest because I could see his back shaking a bit, and I could see movement from her shoulder. I was afraid to see her face. I was afraid she would see mine, just gawping there through the window. And so, since it was not my grief and had not been my operation, since I was feeling no ache from personal loss or personal failure, I walked on and I walked away. I went home, and I never saw any of those people again.

There have been many bloody nights since that one. So that bloodiness has not interrupted my sense of surgery's beauty. And so that I know that the ugliness of that night was not about gore. Nor was it about misdiagnosis, which I have since learned is quite common in cases of leaking aneurysm, and is sometimes unavoidable.

What was awful that night was that, in the name of saving Mr. Cooke's life, in the rush toward an operation that offered the only hope of survival, this man was denied his last minutes of liberty. The short time he had left was taken from him, minutes he would probably have spent holding his wife's hand as I had seen him do so easily when I had been talking to them earlier that night. Instead, he was rushed off, to meet a terrified end in a strange and brutal place at the hands of people who—though they aimed to be saviors—became his executioners.

I still see the beauty of surgery all around me when I'm at work. In clear diagnosis. In methodical procedure. In the rudimentary environment of the operating theater. In the rigorous magic performed by surgeons on patients, whose diseases are often cured by going under the knife.

But even the most righteous surgery can be ugly. Even the most necessary operation, in the best hands, can fail. And in the process of acting in patients' best surgical interests, we may sometimes make the final moments of their life more terrible than they would ever have been, had we left them alone to say their farewells uninterfered with, more wholly and with more grace.

Do Not Go Gentle

IRVIN YALOM

I didn't know how to respond. Never before had a patient asked me to be the keeper of love letters. Dave presented his reasons straightforwardly. Sixty-nine-year-old men have been known to die suddenly. In that event, his wife would find the letters and be pained by reading them. There was no one else he could ask to keep them, no friend he had dared tell of this affair. His lover, Soraya? Thirty years dead. She had died while giving birth. Not his child, Dave was quick to add. God knows what had happened to his letters to her!

"What do you want me to do with them?" I asked.

"Nothing. Do nothing at all. Just keep them."

"When was the last time you read them?"

"I haven't read them for at least twenty years."

"They seem like such a hot potato," I ventured. "Why keep them at all?"

Dave looked at me incredulously. I think a shiver of doubt went through him. Was I really that stupid? Had he made a mistake in thinking I was sensitive enough to help him? After a few seconds, he said, "I'll never destroy those letters."

These words had an edge to them, the first signs of strain in the relationship we had been forming over the past six months. My comment had been a blunder, and I retreated to a more conciliatory, open-ended line of questioning. "Dave, tell me some more about the letters and what they mean to you."

Dave began to talk about Soraya, and in a few minutes the tension had gone and his self-assured, easy jauntiness returned. He had met her while he was managing a branch of an American company in Beirut. She was the most beautiful woman he had ever conquered. *Conquer* was his word. Dave always surprised me with such statements, part ingenuousness, part cynicism. How could he say *conquer*? Was he even less self-aware than I had thought? Or was it possible that he was far ahead of me, and mocked himself—and me, too—with subtle irony?

He had loved Soraya—or, at least, she was the only one of his lovers (and they had been legion) to whom he had ever said "I love you." He and Soraya had a deliciously clandestine affair for four years. (Not delicious *and* clandestine but *deliciously clandestine,* for secrecy—and I shall say more about this shortly—was the axis of Dave's personality around which all else rotated. He was aroused by, compelled by, secrecy, and often courted it at great personal expense. Many relationships, especially those with his two ex-wives and his current wife, had been twisted and torn by his unwillingness to be open or straight about anything.)

After four years, Dave's company transferred him to another part of the world, and for the next six years until her death Dave and Soraya saw each other only four times. But they corresponded almost daily. He had kept Soraya's letters (numbering in the hundreds) well hidden. Sometimes he put them in a file cabinet in quirky categories (under G for guilty, or D for depression—that is, to be read when deeply depressed).

Once, for three years, he had stored them in a safe-deposit box. I wondered, but did not ask, about the relationship between his wife and the key to that safe-deposit box. Knowing his penchant for secrecy and intrigue, I could imagine what would happen: he would accidentally let his wife see the key, and then devise an obviously false cover story to churn her curiosity; then, as she grew anxious and inquisitive, he would proceed to despise her for snooping and for constricting him by her unseemly suspiciousness. Dave had frequently enacted that type of scenario.

"Now I'm getting more and more nervous about Soraya's letters, and I wondered if you'd keep them. It's just that simple."

We both looked at his large briefcase bulging with words of love from Soraya—the long-dead, dear Soraya whose brain and mind had vanished, whose scattered DNA molecules had drained back into the basin of earth, and who, for thirty years, had not thought of Dave or anything else.

I wondered whether Dave could step back and become witness to himself. To see how ludicrous, how pathetic, how idolatrous he was—an old man, stumbling toward death, comforted only by a clutch of letters, a marching banner proclaiming that he had loved and been loved once, thirty years before. Would it help Dave to see that image? Could I help him assume the "witness to himself" posture without his feeling that I was demeaning both him and the letters?

To my mind, "good" therapy (which I equate with deep, or penetrating, therapy, not with efficient or even, I am pained to say, helpful therapy) conducted with a "good" patient is at bottom a truth-seeking venture. My quarry when I was a novitiate was the truth of the past, to trace all of a life's coordinates and, thereby, to locate and to explain a person's current life, pathology, motivation, and actions.

I used to be so sure. What arrogance! And *now* what

kind of truth was I stalking? I think my quarry is illusion. I war against magic. I believe that, though illusion often cheers and comforts, it ultimately and invariably weakens and constricts the spirit.

But there is timing and judgment. Never take away anything if you have nothing better to offer. Beware of stripping a patient who can't bear the chill of reality. And don't exhaust yourself by jousting with religious magic: you're no match for it. The thirst for religion is too strong, its roots too deep, its cultural reinforcement too powerful.

Yet I am not without faith, my Hail Mary being the Socratic incantation "The unexamined life is not worth living." But that was not Dave's faith. So I curbed my curiosity. Dave scarcely wondered about the ultimate meaning of his clutch of letters and now, tight and brittle, he would not be receptive to such an inquiry. Nor would it be helpful—now or probably ever.

Besides, my questions had a hollow ring. I saw much of myself in Dave, and there are limits to my hypocrisy. I, too, had my sack of letters from a long-lost love. I, too, had them cutely hidden away (in my system, under B for *Bleak House*, my favorite Dickens novel, to be read when life was at its bleakest). I, too, had never reread the letters. Whenever I tried, they brought pain, not comfort. They had lain there untouched for fifteen years, and I, too, could not destroy them.

Were I my own patient (or my own therapist), I would say, "Imagine the letters gone, destroyed, or lost. What would you feel? Plunge into that feeling, explore it." But I could not. Often I thought of burning them, but that thought always evoked an inexpressible ache. My great interest in Dave, my surge of curiosity and fascination, I knew whence it came: I was asking Dave to do my work for me. Or *our* work for *us*.

From the outset, I had felt drawn to Dave. At our first session six months before, I had asked him, after a few pleasantries, "What ails?"

He responded, "I can't get it up anymore!"

I was astonished. I remember looking at him—his tall, lean, athletic body, his full head of glistening black hair, and his lively elfish eyes belying his sixty-nine years—and thinking, "*Chapeaux!*" ("Hats off!"). My father had done his first coronary at forty-eight. I hoped that when I was sixty-nine I'd be sufficiently alive and vital to worry about "getting it up."

Dave and I both had a proclivity to sexualize much in our environment. I contained it better than he, and had long since learned to prevent it from dominating my life. I also did not share Dave's passion for secrecy, and have many friends, including my wife, with whom I share everything.

Back to the letters. What should I do? Should I keep Dave's letters? Well, why not? After all, was it not an auspicious sign that he was willing to trust me? He had never been able to confide much in anyone, and certainly not in a male. Although impotence had been his explicit reason for choosing to see me, I felt that the real task of therapy was to improve the way he related to others. A trusting, confiding relationship is a prerequisite for any therapy and, in Dave's, might be instrumental in changing his pathological need for secrecy. Keeping the letters would forge a bond of trust between us.

Perhaps the letters might give me additional leverage. I had never felt that Dave was securely lodged in therapy. We had worked well with his impotence. My tactic had been to focus on the marital discord, and to suggest that impotence was to be expected in a relationship with so much anger and mutual suspicion. Dave, who had been recently married (for the fourth time), described his current marriage in the same way he described his previous marriages: he felt he was in prison, and his wife was a prison guard who listened to his phone conversations and read his mail and personal papers. I had helped him realize that, to the extent that he was in prison, it was a prison of his own construction. *Of course* his wife tried to obtain information. *Of course* she was curious about his actions and correspondence. But it was he who had whetted her curiosity by refusing to share even innocent crumbs of information about his life.

Dave had responded well to this approach, and made impressive attempts to share with his wife more of his life and internal experience. His action broke the vicious circle, his wife softened, his own anger diminished, and his sexual performance improved.

I had turned, now, in treatment, to a consideration of unconscious motivation. What payoff did Dave get from a belief that he was imprisoned by a woman? What fueled his passion for secrecy? What had prevented him from forming even one intimate, nonsexualized relationship with either man or woman? What had happened to his cravings for closeness? Could these cravings, even now at sixty-nine, be excavated, reanimated, and realized?

But these seemed more *my* project than Dave's. I suspected that, in part, he agreed to examine unconscious motivations simply to humor me. He liked to talk to me, but I believe that the primary attraction was the opportunity to reminisce, to keep alive the halcyon days of sexual triumph. My connection with him felt tentative. I always felt that if I probed too far, ranged too close to his anxiety, he would simply disappear—fail to show up for his next appointment, and I would never be able to contact him again.

If I kept the letters, they could act as a guyline: he couldn't simply float away and disappear. At the very least, he would have to be up front about terminating: he'd have to face me and request the letters back.

Besides, I felt I *had* to accept the letters. Dave was so hypersensitive. How could I reject the letters without his feeling I was rejecting him? He was also highly judgmental. A mistake would be fatal: he rarely gave people a second chance.

Yet I was uncomfortable with Dave's request. I began to think of good reasons *not* to accept his letters. I would be making a pact with his shadow—an alliance with pathology. There was something conspiratorial about the request. We'd be relating together as two bad little boys. Could I build a solid therapeutic relationship on such insubstantial foundations?

My idea that keeping the letters would make it harder for Dave to terminate therapy was, I realized quickly, nonsense. I dismissed this angle as being just that—an angle, one of my dumb, harebrained, manipulative ploys that always backfire. Angles or gimmicks were not going to help Dave relate to others directly and authentically: I had to model straightforward, honest behavior.

Besides, if he wanted to stop therapy, he'd find a way to get the letters back. I recall a patient I saw twenty years ago whose therapy was pockmarked with duplicity. She was a multiple personality whose two personae (whom I shall call Blush and Brazen) waged a deceitful war against each other. The person I treated was Blush, a constricted, prudish young thing, while Brazen, whom I rarely encountered, referred to herself as a "sexual supermarket" and dated the king of

California pornography. Blush often "awoke" surprised to find that Brazen had emptied her bank account and bought sexy gowns, red lace underwear, and airline tickets for jaunts to Tijuana and Las Vegas. One day, Blush was alarmed to find an around-the-world airline ticket on her dresser, and thought that she could prevent the trip by locking up all of Brazen's sexy clothing in my office. Somewhat bemused and willing to try anything once, I agreed and stored her clothes under my desk. A week later, I arrived at work one morning to find my door broken open, my office rifled, and the clothes gone. Gone was also my patient. I never saw Blush (or Brazen) again.

Suppose Dave did die on me? However good his health, he *was* sixty-nine. People *do* die at sixty-nine. What would I do with the letters then? Besides, where in the hell would I store them? Those letters must weigh ten pounds. I imagined, for a moment, interring them together with mine. They might, if discovered, provide me some cover.

But the really major problem with keeping the letters had to do with group therapy. Several weeks before, I had suggested to Dave that he enter a therapy group, and over the past three sessions we had discussed this at great length. His penchant for concealment, his sexualization of all transactions with women, his fear and distrust of all men—all of these traits, it seemed to me, were excellent issues to work on in group therapy. Reluctantly, he had agreed to begin my therapy group, and our session that day was to be our last individual meeting.

Dave's request for me to keep the letters had to be seen in this context. First, it was entirely possible that the imminent transfer to the group was the factor behind his request. No doubt he regretted losing his exclusive relationship with me and resented the idea of sharing me with the group members. Asking me to keep the letters might, thus, be a way of perpetuating our special, and private, relationship.

I tried very, very delicately to express that idea, in order not to provoke Dave's exquisite sensitivity. I was careful not to demean the letters by suggesting he was using them as a means to an end. I was also careful to avoid sounding as though I were minutely scrutinizing our relationship: this was a time to nurture its growth.

Dave, being a person who needed extensive time in therapy simply to learn how to use it, scoffed at my interpretation instead of considering whether there was any truth in it. He insisted that he had asked me to keep the letters at this time for one reason only: his wife was now doing a major housecleaning and working her way steadily and surely toward his study, where the letters lay hidden.

I didn't buy his reply, but the moment called for patience, not confrontation. I let it go. I was even more concerned that keeping the letters might ultimately sabotage his work in the therapy group. Group therapy for Dave was, I knew, a high-gain but high-risk venture, and I wanted to facilitate his entry into it.

The benefits might be great. The group could offer Dave a safe community in which he could identify his interpersonal problems and experiment with new behavior. For example, he might reveal more of himself, get closer to other men, relate to women as human beings rather than as sexual parts. Dave unconsciously believed that each of these acts would result in some calamitous event: the group was the ideal arena to disconfirm these assumptions.

Of the many risks, I feared one particular scenario. I imagined that Dave would not only refuse to share important (or trivial) information about himself, but do so in a coy or provocative way. The other group members would proceed to request and then demand more. Dave would respond by sharing less. The group would be angered, and accuse him of playing games with them. Dave would feel hurt and trapped. His suspicions and fears of the group members would be confirmed, and he would drop out of the group, more isolated and discouraged than when he began.

It seemed to me that, if I were to keep the letters, I would be colluding, in a countertherapeutic way, with his penchant for secrecy. Even before starting the group, he would have entered into a conspiracy with me that excluded the other members.

Weighing all these considerations, I finally chose my response.

"I understand why the letters are important to you, Dave, and I also feel good that I'm the one you're willing to entrust with them. However, it's my experience that group therapy works best if everyone in the group, and that includes the group leader, is as open as possible. I really want the group to be helpful to you, and I think it best that we do it this way: I'll be glad to store the letters in a safe, locked place for as long as you wish, provided that you agree to tell the group about our bargain."

Dave looked startled. He hadn't anticipated this. Would he take the leap? He cogitated for a couple of minutes: "I don't know. I'll have to think about it. I'll get back to you." He left my office, his briefcase and homeless letters in tow.

Dave never did get back to me about the letters—at least not in any way I could anticipate. But he did join the group, and attended the first several meetings faithfully. In fact, I was astounded at his enthusiasm: by the fourth meeting, he told us that the group was the high point of his week, and he found himself counting the days till the next session. The reason behind the enthusiasm was, alas, not the lure of self-discovery but the quartet of attractive women members. He focused solely upon them and, we learned later, tried to arrange to meet socially with two of them outside the group.

As I had anticipated, Dave kept himself well concealed in the group and, in fact, received reinforcement for his behavior from another secretive member, a beautiful and proud woman who, like him, looked decades younger than her years. At one meeting, she and Dave were asked to state their ages. Both refused, offering the ingenious dodge that they didn't want to be age-typed. Long ago (when genitals were referred to as "privates"), therapy groups were reluctant to talk about sex. In the last two decades, however, groups talk about sex with some ease, and money has become the private subject. In thousands of group meetings, whose members supposedly bare all, I have yet to hear group members disclose their incomes.

But in Dave's group, the burning secret was age. Dave teased and joked about it, but adamantly refused to state his age: he would not jeopardize his chances of scoring with one of the women in the group. In one meeting, when one of the women members pressed him to tell his age, Dave offered an exchange: his secret, his age, for her home telephone number.

I grew concerned with the amount of resistance in the group. Not only was Dave not seriously working in therapy, but his bantering and flirtatiousness had shifted the entire discourse of the therapy group to a superficial level.

At one meeting, however, the tone turned deeply serious. One woman announced that her boyfriend had just learned he had cancer. She was convinced he was going to die soon, though the doctors claimed that his prognosis was not hopeless despite his debilitated physical condition and his advanced age (he was sixty-three).

I flinched for Dave: that man at the "advanced" age of sixty-three was still six years younger than he. But he didn't bat an eye and, in fact, began to speak in a far more honest fashion.

"Maybe that's something I ought to be talking about in the group. I am very phobic about illness and death. I refuse to see a doctor, a *real* doctor"—gesturing mischievously at me. "My last physical exam was over fifteen years ago."

Another group member: "You look like you're in great shape, Dave, whatever your age."

"Thank you. I work at it. Between swimming, tennis, and walking, I exercise a minimum of two hours a day. Theresa, I feel for you and your boyfriend, but I don't know how to help. I do a lot of thinking about aging and death, but my thoughts are too morbid to talk about. To be honest, I don't even like to visit sick people or listen to talk about illness. The Doc"—again, gesturing at me—"always says I keep things light in the group; maybe that's why!"

"What's why?" I asked.

"Well, if I start being serious here, I'll start talking about how much I hate about growing older, how much I fear death. Some day I'll tell you about my nightmares—maybe."

"You're not the only one who has these fears, Dave. Maybe it would be helpful to find out that everyone's in the same boat."

"No, you're alone in your own boat. That's the most terrible part about dying—you have to do it alone."

Another member: "Even so, even though you're alone in your boat, it's always comforting to see the lights of the other boats bobbing nearby."

As we ended this meeting, I was exceedingly hopeful. It felt like a breakthrough session. Dave was talking about something important, he was moved, he had become real, and the other members responded in kind.

At the next meeting, Dave related a powerful dream he had had the night after the previous session. The dream (recorded verbatim by a student observer):

> Death is all around me. I can smell death. I have a packet with an envelope stuffed inside of it, and the envelope contains something that is immune to death or decay or deterioration. I'm keeping it secret. I go to pick it up and feel it, and suddenly I see that the envelope is empty. I feel very distressed about that and notice that it's been split open. Later I find what I assume was in the envelope on the street, and it is a dirty old shoe with the sole coming off.

The dream floored me. I had often thought about his love letters, and had wondered if I would ever get a chance again to explore their meaning with Dave.

Much as I love to do group therapy, the format has one important drawback for me: it often does not permit the exploration of deeper existential issues. Time and again in a group, I gaze longingly at a beautiful trail that would lead me deep into the interior of a person, but must content myself with the practical (and more helpful) task of clearing away the interpersonal underbrush. Yet I couldn't deny myself this dream; it was the *via regia* into the heart of the forest. Rarely have I ever heard of a dream that so transparently laid out the answer to an unconscious mystery.

Neither Dave nor the group knew what to make of the dream. They floundered for a few minutes, and then I supplied some direction by casually asking Dave whether he had any associations to the dream image of an envelope which he was keeping secret.

I knew I was taking a risk. It would be an error, probably a fatal error, either to force Dave into untimely revealing, or for me to reveal, information he had entrusted to me in our individual work before he started the group. I thought my question was within the margins of safety: I stayed concretely with the dream material, and Dave could easily demur by failing to have pertinent associations.

He gamely proceeded, but not without his usual coyness. He stated that perhaps the dream referred to some letters he had been keeping secret—letters of a "certain relationship." The other members, their curiosity aroused, questioned him until Dave related a few things about his old love affair with Soraya and the problem of finding a suitable resting place for the letters. He did not say that the affair was thirty years over. Nor did he mention his negotiations with me, and my offer to keep the letters for him if he agreed to share all with the group.

The group focused upon the issue of secrecy—not the issue that now most fascinated me, though nonetheless a relevant therapeutic issue. Members wondered about Dave's hiddenness; some could understand his wish to keep the letters secret from his wife, but none could understand his excess of secrecy. For example, why did Dave refuse to tell his wife that he was in therapy? No one bought his lame excuse that, if she knew he was in therapy, she'd be very threatened because she'd think he was there to complain about her, and also she'd make his life miserable by grilling him each week about what he had said in the group.

If he were, indeed, concerned about his wife's peace of mind, they pointed out, look how much more irritating it must be for her not to know where he went each week. Look at all the limp excuses he gave her for leaving the house each week to attend the group (he was retired and had no ongoing business outside the house). And look at the machinations he went through to conceal his therapy-bill payment each month. All this cloak-and-dagger! What for? Even insurance forms had to be sent to his secret post office box number. The members complained, too, of Dave's secretiveness in the group. They felt distanced by his reluctance to trust them. Why did he have to say "letters of a certain relationship" earlier in the meeting?

They confronted him directly: "C'mon, Dave, how much extra would it cost to come out and say 'love letters'?"

The group members, bless their hearts, were doing just what they should have been doing. They chose that part of the dream—the theme of secrecy—that was most relevant to the way Dave related to them, and they whacked away at it beautifully. Though Dave seemed a little anxious, he was refreshingly engaged—no game playing today.

But I got greedy. That dream was pure gold, and I wanted to mine it. "Does anyone have hunches about the rest of the dream?" I asked. "About, for example, the smell of death, and the fact that the envelope contains 'something that is immune to death, decay, or deterioration'?"

The group was silent for a few moments, and then Dave turned to me and said, "What do you think, Doc? I'd be really interested in hearing."

I felt caught. I really couldn't answer without revealing some of the material Dave had shared with me in our individual session. He hadn't, for example, told the group that Soraya had been dead for thirty years, that he was sixty-nine and felt near death, that he had asked me to be the keeper of the letters. Yet, if I revealed these things, Dave would feel betrayed, and would probably leave therapy. Was

I walking into a trap? The only possible way out was to be entirely honest.

I said, "Dave, it's really hard for me to respond to your question. I can't tell you my thoughts about the dream without revealing information you shared with me before you entered the group. I know you're very concerned about your privacy, and I don't want to betray your trust. So what do I do?"

I leaned back, pleased with myself. Excellent technique! Just what I tell my students. If you're caught in a dilemma, or have two strong conflicting feelings, then the best thing you can do is share the dilemma or share both feelings with the patient.

Dave said, "Shoot! Go ahead. I'm paying for your opinion. I have nothing to hide. Anything I've said to you is an open book. I didn't mention our discussion about the letters because I didn't want to compromise you. My request to you and your counteroffer were both a bit wacky."

Now that I had Dave's permission, I proceeded to give the group members, who were by now mystified by our exchange, the relevant background: the great importance of the letters to Dave, Soraya's death thirty years ago, Dave's dilemma about where to store the letters, his request that I store them, and my offer, which he had so far declined, to keep them only if he agreed to inform the group about the entire transaction. I was careful to respect Dave's privacy by not revealing his age or any extraneous material.

Then I turned to the dream. I thought the dream answered the question why the letters were loaded for Dave. And, of course, why my letters were loaded for me. But of my letters I did not speak: there are limits to my courage. Of course, I have my rationalizations. The patients are here for *their* therapy, not mine. Time is valuable in a group—eight patients and only ninety minutes—and is not well spent by the patients listening to the therapist's problems. Patients need to have faith that their therapists face and resolve their personal problems.

But these are indeed rationalizations. The real issue was want of courage. I have erred consistently on the side of too little, rather than too much, self-disclosure; but whenever I have shared a great deal of myself, patients have invariably profited from knowing that I, like them, must struggle with the problem of being human.

The dream, I continued, was a dream about death. It began with "Death is all around me. I can smell death." And the central image was the envelope, an envelope that contained something immune to death and deterioration. What could be clearer? The love letters were an amulet, an instrument of death denial. They warded off aging and kept Dave's passion frozen in time. To be truly loved, to be remembered, to be fused with another forever, is to be imperishable and to be sheltered from the aloneness at the heart of existence.

As the dream continued, Dave saw that the envelope had been slit open and was empty. Why slit open and empty? Perhaps he felt that the letters would lose their power if he shared them with others? There was something patently and privately irrational about the letters' ability to ward off aging and death—a dark magic that evaporates when examined under the cold light of rationality.

A group member asked, "What about the dirty old shoe with the sole coming off?"

I didn't know, but before I could make any response at all, another member said, "That stands for death. The shoe is losing its *soul,* spelled S-O-U-L."

Of course—*soul,* not *sole*! That's beautiful! Why hadn't

I thought of that? I had grasped the first half: I knew that the dirty old shoe represented Dave. On a couple of occasions (for example, that time he asked a woman member forty years younger for her phone number), the group had come close, I thought, to calling Dave a "dirty old man." I winced for him, and was glad that the epithet had not been uttered aloud. But in the group discussion, Dave took it upon himself.

"My God! A dirty old man whose soul is about to leave him. That's me, all right!" He chuckled at his own creation. A lover of words (he spoke several languages), he marveled at the transposition of *soul* and *sole*.

Despite Dave's jocularity, it was apparent he was dealing with very painful material. One of the members asked him to share some more about feeling like a dirty old man. Another asked about what it felt like to reveal the existence of the letters to the group. Would that change his attitude about them? Another one reminded him that everyone faced the prospect of aging and decline, and urged him to share more about this cluster of feelings.

But Dave had closed down. He had done all the work he was to do that day. "I've gotten my money's worth today. I need some time to digest all this. I've taken up seventy-five percent of the meeting already, and I know that others want some time today."

Reluctantly, we left Dave and turned to other matters in the group. We did not know, then, that it was to be a permanent farewell. Dave never returned to another group meeting. (Nor, it turned out, was he willing to resume individual therapy with me or anyone else.)

Everyone, no one more than I, did a great deal of self-questioning. What had we done to drive Dave away? Had we stripped away too much? Had we tried too quickly to make a foolish old man wise? Had I betrayed him? Had I stepped into a trap? Would it have been better not to have spoken of the letters and to have let the dream go? (The dream-interpretative work was successful, but the patient died.)

Perhaps we might have forestalled his departure, but I doubt it. By this time, I was certain that Dave's caginess, his avoidance and denial, would have ultimately led to the same result. I had strongly suspected from the beginning that he would likely drop out of the group. (The fact that I was a better prophet than therapist, however, gave me little solace.)

More than anything, I felt sorrow. Sorrow for Dave, for his isolation, for his clinging to illusion, for his want of courage, for his unwillingness to face the naked, harsh facts of life.

And then I slipped into a reverie about my own letters. What would happen if (I smiled at my "if") I died and they were found? Maybe I *should* give them to Mort or Jay or Pete to store for me? Why do I keep troubling myself about those letters? Why not relieve myself of all this aggravation and burn them? Why not now? Right now! But it hurts to think about it. A stab right through my sternum. But why? Why so much pain about old yellowing letters? I'm going to have to work on this—someday.

The Lost Mariner

OLIVER SACKS

> You have to begin to lose your memory, if only in bits and
> pieces, to realize that memory is what makes our lives.
> Life without memory is no life at all. . . . Our memory is
> our coherence, our reason, our feeling, even our action.
> Without it, we are nothing. (I can only wait for the final
> amnesia, the one that can erase an entire life, as it did my
> mother's. . . .)
>
> *Luis Buñuel*

This moving and frightening segment in Buñuel's recently
translated memoirs raises fundamental questions—clinical,
practical, existential, philosophical: what sort of a life (if
any), what sort of a world, what sort of a self can be preserved in a man who has lost the greater part of his memory,
and, with this, his past, and his moorings in time?

It immediately made me think of a patient of mine in
whom these questions are precisely exemplified: charming,
intelligent, memoryless Jimmie R., who was admitted to our
Home for the Aged near New York City early in 1975, with
a cryptic transfer note saying, "Helpless, demented, confused, and disoriented."

Jimmie was a fine-looking man, with a curly bush of gray
hair, a healthy and handsome forty-nine-year-old. He was
cheerful, friendly, and warm.

"Hiya, Doc!" he said. "Nice morning! Do I take this chair here?" He was a genial soul, very ready to talk and to answer any questions I asked him. He told me his name and birth date, and the name of the little town in Pennsylvania where he was born. He described it in affectionate detail, even drew me a map. He spoke of the houses where his family had lived—he remembered their phone numbers still. He spoke of school and school days, the friends he'd had, and his special fondness for mathematics and science. He talked with enthusiasm of his days in the navy—he was seventeen, had just graduated from high school when he was drafted in 1943. With his good engineering mind, he was a "natural" for radio and electronics, and after a crash course in Texas found himself assistant radio operator on a submarine. He remembered the names of various submarines on which he had served, their missions, where they were stationed, the names of his shipmates. He remembered Morse code, and was still fluent in Morse tapping and touch-typing.

A full and interesting early life, remembered vividly, in detail, with affection. But there, for some reason, his reminiscences stopped. He recalled, and almost relived, his war days and service, the end of the war, and his thoughts for the future. He had come to love the navy, thought he might stay in it. But with the GI Bill, and support, he felt he might do best to go to college. His older brother was in dental school and engaged to a girl, a "real beauty," from California.

With recalling, reliving, Jimmie was full of animation; he did not seem to be speaking of the past but of the present, and I was very struck by the change of tense in his recollections as he passed from his school days to his days in the navy. He had been using the past tense, but now used the present—and (it seemed to me) not just the formal or fictitious present tense of recall, but the actual present tense of immediate experience.

A sudden, improbable suspicion seized me.

"What year is this, Mr. R.?" I asked, concealing my perplexity under a casual manner.

"Forty-five, man. What do you mean?" He went on, "We've won the war, FDR's dead, Truman's at the helm. There are great times ahead."

"And you, Jimmie, how old would you be?"

Oddly, uncertainly, he hesitated a moment, as if engaged in calculation.

"Why, I guess I'm nineteen, Doc. I'll be twenty next birthday."

Looking at the gray-haired man before me, I had an impulse for which I have never forgiven myself—it was, or would have been, the height of cruelty had there been any possibility of Jimmie's remembering it.

"Here," I said, and thrust a mirror toward him. "Look in the mirror and tell me what you see. Is that a nineteen-year-old looking out from the mirror?"

He suddenly turned ashen and gripped the sides of the chair. "Jesus Christ," he whispered. "Christ, what's going on? What's happened to me? Is this a nightmare? Am I crazy? Is this a joke?"—and he became frantic, panicky.

"It's okay, Jim," I said soothingly. "It's just a mistake. Nothing to worry about. Hey!" I took him to the window. "Isn't this a lovely spring day. See the kids there playing baseball?" He regained his color and started to smile, and I stole away, taking the hateful mirror with me.

Two minutes later, I reentered the room. Jimmie was still standing by the window, gazing with pleasure at the kids playing baseball below. He wheeled around as I opened the door, and his face assumed a cheery expression.

"Hiya, Doc!" he said. "Nice morning! You want to talk to me—do I take this chair here?" There was no sign of recognition on his frank, open face.

"Haven't we met before, Mr. R.?" I asked casually.

"No, I can't say we have. Quite a beard you got there. I wouldn't forget *you*, Doc!"

"Why do you call me 'Doc'?"

"Well, you are a doc, ain't you?"

"Yes, but if you haven't met me, how do you know what I am?"

"You *talk* like a doc. I can *see* you're a doc."

"Well, you're right, I am. I'm the neurologist here."

"Neurologist? Hey, there's something wrong with my nerves? And 'here'—where's 'here,' what is this place anyhow?"

"I was just going to ask you—where do you think you are?"

"I see these beds, and these patients everywhere. Looks like a sort of hospital to me. But hell, what would I be doing in a hospital—and with all these old people, years older than me. I feel good, I'm strong as a bull. Maybe I *work* here. . . . Do I work? What's my job? . . . No, you're shaking your head, I see in your eyes I don't work here. If I don't work here, I've been *put* here. Am I a patient, am I sick and don't know it, Doc? It's crazy, it's scary. . . . Is it some sort of joke?"

"You don't know what the matter is? You really don't know? You remember telling me about your childhood, growing up in Pennsylvania, working as a radio operator on submarines? And how your brother is engaged to a girl from California?"

"Hey, you're right. But I didn't tell you that, I never met you before in my life. You must have read all about me in my chart."

"Okay," I said. "I'll tell you a story. A man went to his doctor complaining of memory lapses. The doctor asked him some routine questions, and then said, 'These lapses. What about them?' 'What lapses?' the patient replied."

"So that's my problem," Jimmie laughed. "I kinda thought it was. I do find myself forgetting things, once in a while—things that have just happened. The past is clear, though."

"Will you allow me to examine you, to run over some tests?"

"Sure," he said genially. "Whatever you want."

On intelligence testing he showed excellent ability. He was quick-witted, observant, and logical, and had no difficulty solving complex problems and puzzles—no difficulty, that is, if they could be done quickly. If much time was required, he forgot what he was doing. He was quick and good at tic-tac-toe and checkers, and cunning and aggressive—he easily beat me. But he got lost at chess—the moves were too slow.

Homing in on his memory, I found an extreme and extraordinary loss of recent memory—so that whatever was said or shown or done to him was apt to be forgotten in a few seconds' time. Thus I laid out my watch, my tie, and my glasses on the desk, covered them, and asked him to remember these. Then, after a minute's chat, I asked him what I had put under the cover. He remembered none of them—or indeed that I had even asked him to remember. I repeated the test, this time getting him to write down the names of the three objects; again he forgot, and when I showed him the paper with his writing on it he was astounded, and said he had no recollection of writing anything down, though he acknowledged that it was his own writing, and then got a faint "echo" of the fact that he had written them down.

He sometimes retained faint memories, some dim echo or sense of familiarity. Thus five minutes after I had played tic-tac-toe with him, he recollected that "some doctor" had played this with him "a while back"—whether the "while back" was minutes or months ago he had no idea. He then paused and said, "It could have been you!" When I said it *was* me, he seemed amused. This faint amusement and indifference were very characteristic, as were the involved cogitations to which he was driven by being so disoriented and lost in time. When I asked Jimmie the time of the year, he would immediately look around for some "clue"—I was careful to remove the calendar from my desk—and would "work out" the time of year, roughly, by looking through the window.

It was not, apparently, that he failed to register in memory, but that the memory traces were fugitive in the extreme, and were apt to be effaced within a minute, often less, especially if there were distracting or competing stimuli, while his intellectual and perceptual powers were preserved, and highly superior.

Jimmie's scientific knowledge was that of a bright high school graduate with a penchant for mathematics and science. He was superb at arithmetical (and also algebraic) calculations, but only if they could be done with lightning speed. If there were many steps, too much time involved, he would forget where he was, and even the question. He knew the elements, compared them, and drew the periodic table—but omitted the transuranic elements.

"Is that complete?" I asked when he'd finished.

"It's complete and up-to-date, sir, as far as I know."

"You wouldn't know any elements beyond uranium?"

"You kidding? There's ninety-two elements, and uranium's the last."

I paused and flipped through a *National Geographic* on the table. "Tell me the planets," I said, "and something about them." Unhesitatingly, confidently, he gave me the planets—their names, their discovery, their distance from the sun, their estimated mass, character, and gravity.

"What is this?" I asked, showing him a photo in the magazine I was holding.

"It's the moon," he replied.

"No, it's not," I answered. "It's a picture of the earth taken from the moon."

"Doc, you're kidding! Someone would've had to get a camera up there!"

"Naturally."

"Hell! You're joking—how the hell would you do that?"

Unless he were a consummate actor, a fraud simulating an astonishment he did not feel, this was an utterly convincing demonstration that he was still in the past. His words, his feelings, his innocent wonder, his struggle to make sense of what he saw, were precisely those of an intelligent young man in the 1940s faced with the future, with what had not yet happened, and what was scarcely imaginable. "This more than anything else," I wrote in my notes, "persuades me that his 'cut off' around 1945 is genuine. . . . What I showed him, and told him, produced the authentic amazement which it would have done in an intelligent young man of the pre-Sputnik era."

I found another photo in the magazine and pushed it over to him.

"That's an aircraft carrier," he said. "Real ultramodern design. I never saw one quite like that."

"What's it called?" I asked.

He glanced down, looked baffled, and said, "The *Nimitz*!"

"Something the matter?"

"The hell there is!" he replied hotly. "I know 'em all by name, and I *don't know* a *Nimitz*. . . . Of course there's an Admiral Nimitz, but I never heard they named a carrier after him."

Angrily, he threw the magazine down.

He was becoming fatigued, and somewhat irritable and anxious, under the continuing pressure of anomaly and contradiction, and their fearful implications, to which he could not be entirely oblivious. I had already, unthinkingly, pushed him into panic, and felt it was time to end our session. We wandered over to the window again, and looked down at the sunlit baseball diamond; as he looked, his face relaxed, he forgot the *Nimitz,* the satellite photo, the other horrors and hints, and became absorbed in the game below. Then, as a savory smell drifted up from the dining room, he smacked his lips, said "Lunch!," smiled, and took his leave.

And I myself was wrung with emotion—it was heartbreaking, it was absurd, it was deeply perplexing, to think of his life lost in limbo, dissolving.

"He is, as it were," I wrote in my notes, "isolated in a single moment of being, with a moat or lacuna of forgetting all round him. . . . He is man without a past (or future), stuck in a constantly changing, meaningless moment." And then, more prosaically, "The remainder of the neurological examination is entirely normal. Impression: probably Korsakov's syndrome, due to alcoholic degeneration of the mammillary bodies." My note was a strange mixture of facts and observations, carefully noted and itemized, with irrepressible meditations on what such problems might "mean," in regard to who and what and where this poor man was—whether, indeed, one could speak of an "existence," given so absolute a privation of memory or continuity.

I kept wondering, in this and later notes—unscientifically—about "a lost soul," and how one might establish some continuity, some roots, for he was a man without roots, or rooted only in the remote past.

"Only connect"—but how could he connect, and how could we help him to connect? What was life without connection? "I may venture to affirm," Hume wrote, that we are "nothing but a bundle or collection of different perceptions, which succeed each other with an inconceivable rapidity, and are in a perpetual flux and movement." In some sense, he had been reduced to a "Humean" being—I could not help thinking how fascinated Hume would have been at seeing in Jim his own philosophical "chimera" incarnate, a gruesome reduction of a man to mere disconnected, incoherent flux and change. But a Humean being would not be a being at all, would have no human or personal identity. And Jim was human—all too human—or was he?

Perhaps I could find advice or help in the medical literature—a literature which, for some reason, was largely Russian, from Korsakov's original thesis (Moscow, 1887) about such cases of memory loss, which are still called "Korsakov's syndrome," to A. R. Luria's *Neuropsychology of Memory* (which appeared in translation only a year after I first saw Jim). Korsakov wrote in 1887:

Memory of recent events is disturbed almost exclusively; recent impressions apparently disappear soonest, whereas impressions of long ago are recalled properly, so that the patient's ingenuity, his sharpness of wit, and his resourcefulness remain largely unaffected.

To Korsakov's brilliant but spare observations, almost a century of further research has been added—the richest and deepest, by far, being Luria's. And in Luria's account, science became poetry, and the pathos of radical lostness was evoked. "Gross disturbances of the organization of impressions of events and their sequence in time can always be observed in such patients," he wrote. "In consequence, they lose their integral experience of time and begin to live in a world of isolated impressions." Further, as Luria noted, the eradication of impressions (and their disorder) might spread backward in time—"in the most serious cases . . . even to relatively distant events."

Most of Luria's patients, as described in this book, had massive and serious cerebral tumors, which had the same effects as Korsakov's syndrome, but later spread and were often fatal. Luria included no cases of "simple" Korsakov's syndrome, based on the self-limiting destruction that Korsakov described—neuron destruction, produced by alcohol, in the tiny but crucial mammillary bodies, the rest of the brain being perfectly preserved. And so there was no long-term follow-up of Luria's cases.

I had at first been deeply puzzled, and dubious, even suspicious, about the apparently sharp "cut off" in 1945, a point, a date, which was also symbolically so sharp. After this, I wrote in a subsequent note:

There is a great blank. We do not know what happened then—or subsequently. . . . WE MUST FILL IN THESE "MISSING" YEARS—from his brother, or the Navy, or hospitals he has been to. . . . Could it be that he sustained some massive trauma at this time, some massive cerebral or emotional trauma in combat, in the War, and that *this* may have affected him ever since?

We did various tests on him (EEG, brain scans), and found no evidence of massive brain damage, although atrophy of the tiny mammillary bodies would not show up on such tests. We received reports from the navy indicating that he had remained in the navy until 1965, and that he was perfectly competent at that time.

Then we turned up a short, nasty report from Bellevue Hospital, dated 1971, saying that he was "totally disoriented . . . with an advanced organic brain-syndrome, due to alcohol" (cirrhosis had also developed by this time). From Bellevue, he was sent to a wretched dump in the Village, a so-called nursing home whence he was rescued—lousy, starving—by our Home in 1975.

We located his brother, whom Jim always spoke of as being in dental school and engaged to a girl from California. In fact, he had married the girl from California, had become a father and grandfather, and been in dental practice for thirty years.

Where we had hoped for an abundance of information and feeling from his brother, we received a courteous but somewhat meager letter. It was obvious from reading this—especially reading between the lines—that the brothers had scarcely seen each other since 1943, and had gone separate ways, partly through the vicissitudes of location and profession, and partly through deep (though not estranging) differences of temperament. Jim, it seemed, had never "settled down," was "happy-go-lucky," and "always a drinker." The navy, his brother felt, provided a structure, a life, and the real problems started when he left it, in 1965. Without his habitual structure and anchor, Jim had ceased to work, "gone to pieces," and started to drink heavily. There had been some memory impairment, of the Korsakov type, in the middle and especially the late sixties, but not so severe that Jimmie couldn't "cope" in his nonchalant fashion. But his drinking grew heavier in 1970.

Around Christmas of that year, his brother understood, he had suddenly "blown his top" and become deliriously excited and confused, and it was at this point that he had been taken into Bellevue. During the next month, the excitement and delirium died down, but he was left with deep and bizarre memory lapses, or "deficits," to use the medical jargon. His brother had visited him at this time—they had not met for twenty years—and, to his horror, Jimmie not only failed to recognize him, but said, "Stop joking! You're old enough to be my father. My brother's a young man, just going through dental school."

When I received this information, I was more perplexed still: why did Jimmie not remember his later years in the navy, why did he not recall and organize his memories until 1970? I had not heard then that such patients might have a retrograde amnesia.[1] "I wonder, increasingly," I wrote at this time, "whether there is not an element of hysterical or fugal amnesia—whether he is not in flight from something too awful to recall," and I suggested he be seen by our psychiatrist. Her report was searching and detailed—the examination had included a sodium amytal test, calculated to "release" any memories which might be repressed. She also attempted to hypnotize Jimmie, in the hope of eliciting memories repressed by hysteria—this tends to work well in cases of hysterical amnesia. But it failed because Jim could not be hypnotized, not because of any "resistance," but because of his extreme amnesia, which caused him to lose track of what the hypnotist was saying. (Dr. M. Homonoff, who worked on the amnesia ward at the Boston Veterans Administration hospital, tells me of similar experiences—and of his feeling that this is absolutely characteristic of patients with Korsakov's, as opposed to patients with hysterical amnesia.)

"I have no feeling or evidence," the psychiatrist wrote, "of any hysterical or 'put-on' deficit. He lacks both the means and the motive to make a façade. His memory deficits are organic and permanent and incorrigible, though it is puzzling they should go back so long." Since, she felt, he was "unconcerned . . . manifested no special anxiety . . . constituted no management problem," there was nothing she could offer, or any therapeutic "entrance" or "lever" she could see.

At this point, persuaded that this was, indeed, "pure" Korsakov's, uncomplicated by other factors, emotional or organic, I wrote to Luria and asked his opinion. He spoke in his reply of his patient Bel, whose amnesia had retroactively eradicated ten years.[2] He said he saw no reason why such a retrograde amnesia should not thrust backward decades, or almost a whole lifetime. "I can only wait for the final amnesia," Buñuel writes, "the one that can erase an entire life." But Jimmie's amnesia, for whatever reason, had erased memory and time back to 1945—roughly—and then stopped. Occasionally, he would recall something much later, but the recall was fragmentary and dislocated in time. Once, seeing the word "satellite" in a newspaper headline, he said offhandedly that he'd been involved in a project of satellite tracking while on the ship *Norton Sound,* a memory fragment coming from the early or mid-sixties. But, for all practical purposes, his "cut-off point" was during the mid- (or late) forties, and anything subsequently retrieved was fragmentary, unconnected. This was the case in 1975, and it is still the case now, nine years later.

What could we do? What should we do? "There are no prescriptions in a case like this," Luria wrote.

Do whatever your ingenuity and your heart suggest. There is little or no hope of any recovery in his memory. But a man does not consist of memory alone. He has feeling, will, sensibilities, moral being—matters of which neuro-psychology cannot speak. And it is here, beyond the realm of an impersonal psychology, that you may find ways to touch him, and change him. And the circumstances of your work especially allow this, for you work in a Home, which is like a little world, quite different from the clinics and institutions where I work. Neuropsychologically, there is little or nothing you can do; but in the realm of the Individual, there may be much you can do.

Luria mentioned his patient Kur as manifesting a rare self-awareness, in which hopelessness was mixed with an odd equanimity. ("I have no memory of the present," Kur would say. "I do not know what I have just done or from where I have just come. . . . I can recall my past very well, but I have no memory of my present.") When asked whether he had ever seen the person testing him, he said, "I cannot say yes or no, I can neither affirm nor deny that I have seen you." This was sometimes the case with Jimmie; and, like Kur, who stayed many months in the same hospital, Jimmie began to form "a sense of familiarity"; he slowly learned his way around the Home—the whereabouts of the dining room, his own room, the elevators, the stairs—and in some sense recognized some of the staff, although he confused them, and perhaps had to do so, with people from the past. He soon became fond of the nursing Sister in the Home; he recognized her voice, her footfalls, immediately, but would always say that she had been a fellow pupil at his high school, and was greatly surprised when I addressed her as "Sister." "Gee!" he exclaimed, "the damnedest things happen. I'd never have guessed you'd become a religious, Sister!"

Since he's been at our Home—that is, since early 1975—Jim has never been able to identify anyone in it consistently. The only person he truly recognizes is his brother, whenever he visits from California. These meetings are deeply emotional and moving to observe—the only truly emotional meetings Jim has. He loves his brother, he recognizes him, but he cannot understand why he looks so old: "Guess some people age fast," he says. Actually, his brother looks much younger than his age, and has the sort of face and build that change little with the years. These then are true meetings, Jim's only connection of past and present, yet they do nothing to provide any sense of history or continuity. If anything, they emphasize—at least to his brother, and to others who see them together—that Jim still lives, is fossilized, in the past.

All of us, at first, had high hopes of helping Jim—he was so personable, so likable, so quick and intelligent, it was difficult to believe that he might be beyond help. But none of us had ever encountered, even imagined, such a power of amnesia, the possibility of a pit into which everything, every experience, every event, would fathomlessly drop, a bottomless memory-hole that would engulf the whole world.

I suggested, when I first saw him, that he should keep a diary, and be encouraged to keep notes every day of his experiences, his feelings, thoughts, memories, reflections. These attempts were foiled, at first, by his continually losing the diary: it had to be attached to him—somehow. But this too failed to "work": he dutifully kept a brief daily notebook, but could not recognize his earlier entries in it. He does recognize his own writing, and style, and is always astounded to find that he wrote something the day before.

Astounded—and indifferent—for he was a man who, in effect, had no "day before." His entries remained unconnected and unconnecting, and had no power to provide any sense of time or continuity. Moreover, they were trivial— "Eggs for breakfast," "Watched ballgame on TV"—and never touched the depths. But were there depths in this unmemoried man, depths of an abiding feeling and thinking, or had he been reduced to a sort of Humean drivel, a mere succession of unrelated impressions and events?

Jimmie both was and wasn't aware of this deep, tragic loss in himself, loss *of* himself. (If a man has lost a leg or an eye, he knows he has lost a leg or an eye; but if he has lost a self—himself—he cannot know it, because he is no longer there to know it.) Therefore I could not question him intellectually about such matters.

He had originally professed bewilderment at finding himself amid patients, when, as he said, he himself didn't feel ill. But what, we wondered, did he feel? He was strongly built and fit, he had a sort of animal strength and energy, but also a strange inertia, passivity, and (as everyone remarked) "unconcern"; he gave all of us an overwhelming sense of "something missing," although this, if he realized it, was itself accepted with an odd "unconcern." One day, I asked him not about his memory, or past, but about the simplest and most elemental feelings of all:

"How do you feel?"

"How do I feel," he repeated, and scratched his head. "I cannot say I feel ill. But I cannot say I feel well. I cannot say I feel anything at all."

"Are you miserable?" I continued.

"Can't say I am."

"Do you enjoy life?"

"I can't say I do."

I hesitated, fearing that I was going too far, that I might be stripping a man down to some hidden, unacknowledge-able, unbearable despair.

"You don't enjoy life," I repeated, hesitating somewhat. "How then *do* you feel about life?"

"I can't say that I feel anything at all."

"You feel alive, though?"

" 'Feel alive' . . . Not really. I haven't felt alive for a very long time."

His face wore a look of infinite sadness and resignation.

Later, having noted his aptitude for, and pleasure in, quick games and puzzles, and their power to "hold" him, at least while they lasted, and to allow, for a while, a sense of companionship and competition—he had not complained of loneliness, but he looked so alone; he never expressed sadness, but he looked so sad—I suggested he be brought into our recreation programs at the Home. This worked better—better than the diary. He would become keenly and briefly involved in games, but soon they ceased to offer any challenge: he solved all the puzzles, and could solve them easily; and he was far better and sharper than anyone else at games. And as he found this out, he grew fretful and restless again, and wandered the corridors, uneasy and bored and with a sense of indignity—games and puzzles were for chil-dren, a diversion. Clearly, passionately, he wanted some-thing to do: he wanted to do, to be, to feel—and could not; he wanted sense, he wanted purpose—in Freud's words, "work and love."

Could he do "ordinary" work? He had "gone to pieces," his brother said, when he ceased to work in 1965. He had two striking skills—Morse code and touch-typing. We could not use Morse, unless we invented a use; but good typing we could use, if he could recover his old skills—and this would be real work, not just a game. Jim soon did recover his old skills and came to type very quickly—he could not do it slowly—and found in this some of the challenge and satisfaction of a job. But still this was superficial tapping and typing; it was trivial, it did not touch the depths. And what he typed, he typed mechanically—he could not hold the thought—the short sentences following one another in a meaningless order.

One tended to speak of him, instinctively, as a spiritual casualty—a "lost soul": was it possible that he had really been "de-souled" by a disease? "Do you think he *has* a soul?" I once asked the Sisters. They were outraged by my question, but could see why I asked it. "Watch Jimmie in chapel," they said, "and judge for yourself."

I did, and I was moved, profoundly moved and impressed, because I saw here an intensity and steadiness of attention and concentration that I had never seen before in him, or conceived him capable of. I watched him pray, I watched him at Mass, I watched him kneel and take the Sacrament on his tongue, and could not doubt the fullness and totality of Communion, the perfect alignment of his spirit with the spirit of the Mass. Fully, intensely, quietly, in the quietude of absolute concentration and attention, he entered and partook of the Holy Communion. He was wholly held, absorbed, by a feeling. There was no forgetting, no Korsakov's then, nor did it seem possible or imaginable that there should be; for he was no longer at the mercy of a faulty and fallible mechanism—that of meaningless sequences and memory traces—but was absorbed in an act, an act of his whole being, which carried feeling and meaning in an organic continuity and unity, a continuity and unity so seamless it could not permit any break.

Clearly, Jim found himself, found continuity and reality,

in the absoluteness of spiritual attention and act. The Sisters were right—he did find his soul here. And so was Luria, whose words now came back to me: "A man does not consist of memory alone. He has feeling, will, sensibility, moral being. . . . It is here . . . you may touch him, and see a profound change." Memory, mental activity, mind alone, could not hold him; but moral attention and action could hold him completely.

But perhaps "moral" was too narrow a word—for the aesthetic and dramatic were equally involved. Seeing Jim in the chapel opened my eyes to other realms where the soul is called on, and held, and stilled, in attention and communion. The same depth of absorption and attention was to be seen in relation to music and art: he had no difficulty, I noticed, "following" music or simple dramas, for every moment in music and art refers to, contains, other moments. He likes gardening, and has taken over some of the work in our garden. At first, he greeted the garden each day as new, but for some reason this has become more familiar to him than the inside of the Home. He almost never gets lost or disoriented in the garden now; he patterns it, I think, on loved and remembered gardens from his youth in Pennsylvania.

Jim, who was so lost in extensional "spatial" time, was perfectly organized in Bergsonian "intentional" time; what was fugitive, unsustainable, as formal structure, was perfectly stable, perfectly held, as art or will. Moreover, there was something that endured and survived. If Jim was briefly "held" by a task or puzzle or game or calculation, held in the purely mental challenge of these, he would fall apart as soon as they were done, into the abyss of his nothingness, his amnesia. But if he were held in emotional and spiritual attention—in the contemplation of nature or art, in listening to music, in taking part in the Mass in chapel—the attention, its "mood," its quietude, would persist for a while, and there would be in him a pensiveness and peace we rarely, if ever, saw during the rest of his life at the Home.

I have known Jim now for nine years—and neuropsychologically, he has not changed in the least. He still has the severest, most devastating Korsakov's, cannot remember isolated items for more than a few seconds, and has a dense amnesia going back to 1945. But humanly, spiritually, he is at times a different man altogether—no longer fluttering, restless, bored, and lost, but deeply attentive to the beauty and "soul" of the world, rich in all the Kierkegaardian categories—the aesthetic, the moral, the religious, the dramatic. I had wondered, when I first met him, if he were not condemned to a sort of Humean froth, a meaningless fluttering on the surface of life, and whether there was any way of transcending the incoherence of his Humean disease. Empirical science told me there was not—but empirical science, empiricism, takes no account of the soul, no account of what constitutes and determines personal being. Perhaps there is a philosophical as well as a clinical lesson here: that in Korsakov's, or dementia, or other such catastrophes, however great the organic damage and Humean dissolution, there remains the undiminished possibility of reintegration by art, by communion, by touching the human spirit; and this can be preserved in what seems at first a hopeless state of neurological devastation.

Notes

1. My ignorance. I know now that retrograde amnesia, to some degree, is very common, if not universal, in cases of Korsakov's. The classical Korsakov's syndrome—a profound and permanent, but "pure," devastation of memory caused by alcoholic destruction of the mammil-

lary bodies—is rare, even among very heavy drinkers. One may, of course, see Korsakov's syndrome with other pathologies, as in Luria's patients with tumors. A particularly fascinating case of an acute (and mercifully transient) Korsakov's syndrome has been well described only very recently in the so-called transient global amnesia (TGA) which may occur with head injuries, or impaired blood supply to the brain. Here, for a few minutes or hours, a severe and singular amnesia may occur, even though the patient may continue to drive a car or, perhaps, to carry on medical or editorial duties, in a mechanical way. But under this fluency lies a profound amnesia—every sentence uttered being forgotten as soon as it is said, everything forgotten within a few minutes of being seen, though long-established memories and routines may be perfectly preserved.

Further, there may be a profound *retrograde* amnesia in such cases. My colleague Dr. Leon Protass tells me of such a case seen by him recently, in which the patient, a highly intelligent man, was unable for some hours to remember his wife or children, to remember that he had a wife or children. In effect, he lost thirty years of his life—though, fortunately, for only a few hours.

Recovery from such attacks is prompt and complete—yet they are, in a sense, the most horrifying of "little strokes" in their power absolutely to annul or obliterate decades of richly lived, richly achieving, richly memoried life. The horror, typically, is felt only by others—the patient, unaware, amnesiac for his amnesia, may continue what he is doing, quite unconcerned, and only discover later that he lost not only a day (as is common with ordinary alcoholic "blackouts"), but half a lifetime, and never knew it. The fact that one can lose the greater part of a lifetime has peculiar, uncanny horror.

There could be only one thing worse—and that would be to lose one's *entire* lifetime. My friend Dr. Isabelle Rapin, author of *Children with Brain Dysfunction: Neurology, Cognition, Language, and Behavior,* tells me that very rarely, in consequence of certain brain tumors or degenerative diseases, children may develop a severe Korsakov's syndrome. If this happens, it has been thought, they risk losing their childhood and even their infancy from a retrograde amnesia which may extend back to birth. Such children may not only become as helpless as newborns but may also become deeply "autistic" as they lose and forget all human relationships, even the most elemental—the memory of mother love.

In adulthood, life, higher life, may be brought to a premature end by strokes, senility, brain injuries, etc., but there usually remains the consciousness of life lived, of one's past. This is usually felt as a sort of compensation: "At least I lived fully, tasting life to the full, before I was brain-injured, stricken, etc." This sense of "the life lived before," which may be either a consolation or a torment, is precisely what is taken away in retrograde amnesia. The "final amnesia, the one that can erase an entire life" that Buñuel speaks of, may occur, perhaps, in a terminal dementia, but not, in my experience, suddenly, in consequence of a stroke. But there is a different, yet comparable, sort of amnesia, which can occur suddenly—different in that it is not "global" but "modality-specific."

Thus, in one patient under my care, a sudden thrombosis in the posterior circulation of the brain caused the immediate death of the visual parts of the brain. Forthwith, this patient became completely blind—*but did not know it*. He looked blind—but he made no complaints. Questioning and testing showed, beyond doubt, that not only was he centrally or "cortically" blind, but he had lost all visual images and memories, lost them totally—yet had no sense of any loss. Indeed, he had lost the very idea of "seeing"—and was not only unable to describe anything visually, but bewildered when I used words such as "seeing" and "light." He had become, in essence, a nonvisual being. His entire lifetime of seeing, of visuality, had, in effect, been stolen. His whole visual life had, indeed, been erased—and erased permanently in the instant of his stroke. Such a visual amnesia, and (so to speak) blindness to the blindness, amnesia for the amnesia, is in effect a "total" Korsakov's, confined to visuality.

A still more limited, but nonetheless total, amnesia may be displayed with regard to particular forms of perception. Thus, in one patient whose history I have already described ("The Man Who Mistook His Wife for a Hat," *London Review of Books,* May 1983), there was an absolute "prosopagnosia," or agnosia for faces. This patient was not only unable to recognize faces, but unable to imagine or remember any faces—he had indeed lost the very idea of a "face," as my more afflicted patient had lost the very idea of "seeing" or "light." Such syndromes were described by Anton in the 1890s. But the implication of these syndromes—Korsakov's and Anton's—what they entail and must entail for the "world," the lives, the identities, of affected patients, has been scarcely touched on even to this day.

2. See A. R. Luria, *The Neuropsychology of Memory* (New York: Halsted Press, 1976).

The Learning Curve

ATUL GAWANDE

The patient needed a central line. "Here's your chance," S., the chief resident, said. I had never done one before. "Get set up and then page me when you're ready to start."

It was my fourth week in surgical training. The pockets of my short white coat bulged with patient printouts, laminated cards with instructions for doing CPR and reading EKGs and using the dictation system, two surgical handbooks, a stethoscope, wound-dressing supplies, meal tickets, a penlight, scissors, and about a dollar in loose change. As I headed up the stairs to the patient's floor, I rattled.

This will be good, I tried to tell myself: my first real procedure. The patient—fiftyish, stout, taciturn—was recovering from abdominal surgery he'd had about a week earlier. His bowel function hadn't yet returned, and he was unable to eat. I explained to him that he needed intravenous nutrition and that this required a "special line" that would go into his chest. I said that I would put the line in him while he was in his bed, and that it would involve my numbing a spot on his chest with a local anesthetic, and then threading the line in. I did not say that the line was eight inches long and would go into his vena cava, the main blood vessel to his heart. Nor did I say how tricky the procedure could be. There were "slight risks" involved, I said, such as bleeding and lung collapse; in experienced hands, complications of this sort occur in fewer than one case in a hundred.

But, of course, mine were not experienced hands. And the disasters I knew about weighed on my mind: the woman who had died within minutes from massive bleeding when a resident lacerated her vena cava; the man whose chest had to be opened because a resident lost hold of a wire inside the line, which then floated down to the patient's heart; the man who had a cardiac arrest when the procedure put him into ventricular fibrillation. I said nothing of such things, naturally, when I asked the patient's permission to do his line. He said, "OK."

I had seen S. do two central lines; one was the day before, and I'd attended to every step. I watched how she set out her instruments and laid her patient down and put a rolled towel between his shoulder blades to make his chest arch out. I watched how she swabbed his chest with antiseptic, injected lidocaine, which is a local anesthetic, and then, in full sterile garb, punctured his chest near his clavicle with a fat three-inch needle on a syringe. The patient hadn't even flinched. She told me how to avoid hitting the lung ("Go in at a steep angle," she'd said. "Stay *right* under the clavicle"), and how to find the subclavian vein, a branch to the vena cava lying atop the lung near its apex ("Go in at a steep angle. Stay *right* under the clavicle"). She pushed the needle in almost all the way. She drew back on the syringe. And she was in. You knew because the syringe filled with maroon blood. ("If it's bright red, you've hit an artery," she said. "That's not good.") Once you have the tip of this needle poking in the vein, you somehow have to widen the hole in the vein wall, fit the catheter in, and snake it in the right direction—down to the heart, rather than up to the

brain—all without tearing through vessels, lung, or anything else.

To do this, S. explained, you start by getting a guide wire
in place. She pulled the syringe off, leaving the needle in.
Blood flowed out. She picked up a two-foot-long twenty-
gauge wire that looked like the steel D string of an electric
guitar, and passed nearly its full length through the needle's
bore, into the vein, and onward toward the vena cava.
"Never force it in," she warned, "and never, ever let go of
it." A string of rapid heartbeats fired off on the cardiac
monitor, and she quickly pulled the wire back an inch. It
had poked into the heart, causing momentary fibrillation.
"Guess we're in the right place," she said to me quietly.
Then to the patient: "You're doing great. Only a few minutes now." She pulled the needle out over the wire and
replaced it with a bullet of thick, stiff plastic, which she
pushed in tight to widen the vein opening. She then removed
this dilator and threaded the central line—a spaghetti-thick,
flexible yellow plastic tube—over the wire until it was all
the way in. Now she could remove the wire. She flushed the
line with a heparin solution and sutured it to the patient's
chest. And that was it.

Today, it was my turn to try. First, I had to gather supplies—a central-line kit, gloves, gown, cap, mask, lidocaine—
which took me forever. When I finally had the stuff together,
I stopped for a minute outside the patient's door, trying to
recall the steps. They remained frustratingly hazy. But I
couldn't put it off any longer. I had a page-long list of other
things to get done: Mrs. A needed to be discharged; Mr. B
needed an abdominal ultrasound arranged; Mrs. C needed
her skin staples removed. And every fifteen minutes or so I
was getting paged with more tasks: Mr. X was nauseated

and needed to be seen; Miss Y's family was here and needed "someone" to talk to them; Mr. Z needed a laxative. I took a deep breath, put on my best don't-worry-I-know-what-I'm-doing look, and went in.

I placed the supplies on a bedside table, untied the patient's gown, and laid him down flat on the mattress, with his chest bare and his arms at his sides. I flipped on a fluorescent overhead light and raised his bed to my height. I paged S. I put on my gown and gloves and, on a sterile tray, laid out the central line, the guide wire, and other materials from the kit. I drew up five cc's of lidocaine in a syringe, soaked two sponge sticks in the yellow-brown Betadine, and opened up the suture packaging.

S. arrived. "What's his platelet count?"

My stomach knotted. I hadn't checked. That was bad: too low and he could have a serious bleed from the procedure. She went to check a computer. The count was acceptable.

Chastened, I started swabbing his chest with the sponge sticks. "Got the shoulder roll underneath him?" S. asked. Well, no, I had forgotten that, too. The patient gave me a look. S., saying nothing, got a towel, rolled it up, and slipped it under his back for me. I finished applying the antiseptic and then draped him so that only his right upper chest was exposed. He squirmed a bit beneath the drapes. S. now inspected my tray. I girded myself.

"Where's the extra syringe for flushing the line when it's in?" Damn. She went out and got it.

I felt for my landmarks. *Here?* I asked with my eyes, not wanting to undermine the patient's confidence any further. She nodded. I numbed the spot with lidocaine. ("You'll feel a stick and a burn now, sir.") Next, I took the three-inch needle in hand and poked it through the skin. I advanced it slowly and uncertainly, a few millimeters at a time. This is a big goddam needle, I kept thinking. I couldn't believe I was sticking it into someone's chest. I concentrated on maintaining a steep angle of entry, but kept spearing his clavicle instead of slipping beneath it.

"Ow!" he shouted.

"Sorry," I said. S. signaled with a kind of surfing hand gesture to go underneath the clavicle. This time, it went in. I drew back on the syringe. Nothing. She pointed deeper. I went in deeper. Nothing. I withdrew the needle, flushed out some bits of tissue clogging it, and tried again.

"*Ow!*"

Too steep again. I found my way underneath the clavicle once more. I drew the syringe back. Still nothing. He's too obese, I thought. S. slipped on gloves and a gown. "How about I have a look?" she said. I handed her the needle and stepped aside. She plunged the needle in, drew back on the syringe, and, just like that, she was in. "We'll be done shortly," she told the patient.

She let me continue with the next steps, which I bumbled through. I didn't realize how long and floppy the guide wire was until I pulled the coil out of its plastic sleeve, and, putting one end of it into the patient, I very nearly contaminated the other. I forgot about the dilating step until she reminded me. Then, when I put in the dilator, I didn't push quite hard enough, and it was really S. who pushed it all the way in. Finally, we got the line in, flushed it, and sutured it in place.

Outside the room, S. said that I could be less tentative the next time, but that I shouldn't worry too much about how things had gone. "You'll get it," she said. "It just takes practice." I wasn't so sure. The procedure remained wholly mysterious to me. And I could not get over the idea of jabbing a needle into someone's chest so deeply and so blindly. I awaited the X-ray afterward with trepidation. But it came back fine: I had not injured the lung and the line was in the right place.

Not everyone appreciates the attractions of surgery. When you are a medical student in the operating room for the first time, and you see the surgeon press the scalpel to someone's body and open it like a piece of fruit, you either shudder in horror or gape in awe. I gaped. It was not just the blood and guts that enthralled me. It was also the idea that a person, a mere mortal, would have the confidence to wield that scalpel in the first place.

There is a saying about surgeons: "Sometimes wrong; never in doubt." This is meant as a reproof, but to me it seemed their strength. Every day, surgeons are faced with uncertainties. Information is inadequate; the science is ambiguous; one's knowledge and abilities are never perfect. Even with the simplest operation, it cannot be taken for granted that a patient will come through better off—or even alive. Standing at the operating table, I wondered how the surgeon knew that all the steps would go as planned, that bleeding would be controlled and infection would not set in and organs would not be injured. He didn't, of course. But he cut anyway.

Later, while still a student, I was allowed to make an incision myself. The surgeon drew a six-inch dotted line with a marking pen across an anesthetized patient's abdomen and then, to my surprise, had the nurse hand me the knife. It was still warm from the autoclave. The surgeon had me stretch the skin taut with the thumb and forefinger of my free hand. He told me to make one smooth slice down to the fat. I put the belly of the blade to the skin and cut. The experience was odd and addictive, mixing exhilaration from the calculated violence of the act, anxiety about getting it right, and a righteous faith that it was somehow for the person's good. There was also the slightly nauseating feeling of finding that it took more force than I'd realized. (Skin is thick and springy, and on my first pass I did not go nearly deep enough; I had to cut twice to get through.) The moment made me want to be a surgeon—not an amateur handed the knife for a brief moment but someone with the confidence and ability to proceed as if it were routine.

A resident begins, however, with none of this air of mastery—only an overpowering instinct against doing anything like pressing a knife against flesh or jabbing a needle into someone's chest. On my first day as a surgical resident, I was assigned to the emergency room. Among my first patients was a skinny, dark-haired woman in her late twenties who hobbled in, teeth gritted, with a two-foot-long wooden chair leg somehow nailed to the bottom of her foot. She explained that a kitchen chair had collapsed under her and, as she leaped up to keep from falling, her bare foot had stomped down on a three-inch screw sticking out of one of the chair legs. I tried very hard to look like someone who had not got his medical diploma just the week before. Instead, I was determined to be nonchalant, the kind of guy who had seen this sort of thing a hundred times before. I inspected her foot, and could see that the screw was embedded in the bone at the base of her big toe. There was no bleeding and, as far as I could feel, no fracture.

"Wow, that must hurt," I blurted out, idiotically.

The obvious thing to do was give her a tetanus shot and pull out the screw. I ordered the tetanus shot, but I began to have doubts about pulling out the screw. Suppose she bled?

Or suppose I fractured her foot? Or something worse? I excused myself and tracked down Dr. W., the senior surgeon on duty. I found him tending to a car-crash victim. The patient was a mess, and the floor was covered with blood. People were shouting. It was not a good time to ask questions.

I ordered an X-ray. I figured it would buy time and let me check my amateur impression that she didn't have a fracture. Sure enough, getting the X-ray took about an hour, and it showed no fracture—just a common screw embedded, the radiologist said, "in the head of the first metatarsal." I showed the patient the X-ray. "You see, the screw's embedded in the head of the first metatarsal," I said. And the plan? she wanted to know. Ah, yes, the plan.

I went to find Dr. W. He was still busy with the crash victim, but I was able to interrupt to show him the X-ray. He chuckled at the sight of it and asked me what I wanted to do. "Pull the screw out?" I ventured. "Yes," he said, by which he meant "Duh." He made sure I'd given the patient a tetanus shot and then shooed me away.

Back in the examining room, I told her that I would pull the screw out, prepared for her to say something like "You?" Instead she said, "OK, Doctor." At first, I had her sitting on the exam table, dangling her leg off the side. But that didn't look as if it would work. Eventually, I had her lie with her foot jutting off the table end, the board poking out into the air. With every move, her pain increased. I injected a local anesthetic where the screw had gone in and that helped a little. Now I grabbed her foot in one hand, the board in the other, and for a moment I froze. Could I really do this? Who was I to presume?

Finally, I gave her a one-two-three and pulled, gingerly at first and then hard. She groaned. The screw wasn't budging.

I twisted, and abruptly it came free. There was no bleeding.
I washed the wound out, and she found she could walk. I
warned her of the risks of infection and the signs to look for.
Her gratitude was immense and flattering, like the lion's for
the mouse—and that night I went home elated.

In surgery, as in anything else, skill, judgment, and confidence are learned through experience, haltingly and
humiliatingly. Like the tennis player and the oboist and the
guy who fixes hard drives, we need practice to get good at
what we do. There is one difference in medicine, though: we
practice on people.

My second try at placing a central line went no better than
the first. The patient was in intensive care, mortally ill, on a
ventilator, and needed the line so that powerful cardiac
drugs could be delivered directly to her heart. She was also
heavily sedated, and for this I was grateful. She'd be oblivious of my fumbling.

My preparation was better this time. I got the towel roll
in place and the syringes of heparin on the tray. I checked
her lab results, which were fine. I also made a point of drap-
ing more widely, so that if I flopped the guide wire around
by mistake again, it wouldn't hit anything unsterile.

For all that, the procedure was a bust. I stabbed the needle in too shallow and then too deep. Frustration overcame
tentativeness and I tried one angle after another. Nothing
worked. Then, for one brief moment, I got a flash of blood
in the syringe, indicating that I was in the vein. I anchored
the needle with one hand and went to pull the syringe off
with the other. But the syringe was jammed on too tightly,
so that when I pulled it free I dislodged the needle from the
vein. The patient began bleeding into her chest wall. I held

pressure the best I could for a solid five minutes, but still her chest turned black and blue around the site. The hematoma made it impossible to put a line through there anymore. I wanted to give up. But she needed a line and the resident supervising me—a second-year this time—was determined that I succeed. After an X-ray showed that I had not injured her lung, he had me try on the other side, with a whole new kit. I missed again, and he took over. It took him several minutes and two or three sticks to find the vein himself and that made me feel better. Maybe she was an unusually tough case.

When I failed with a third patient a few days later, though, the doubts really set in. Again, it was stick, stick, stick, and nothing. I stepped aside. The resident watching me got it on the next try.

Surgeons, as a group, adhere to a curious egalitarianism. They believe in practice, not talent. People often assume that you have to have great hands to become a surgeon, but it's not true. When I interviewed to get into surgery programs, no one made me sew or take a dexterity test or checked to see if my hands were steady. You do not even need all ten fingers to be accepted. To be sure, talent helps. Professors say that every two or three years they'll see someone truly gifted come through a program—someone who picks up complex manual skills unusually quickly, sees tissue planes before others do, anticipates trouble before it happens. Nonetheless, attending surgeons say that what's most important to them is finding people who are conscientious, industrious, and boneheaded enough to keep at practicing this one difficult thing day and night for years on end. As a former residency director put it to me, given a choice between a Ph.D. who had cloned a gene and a sculptor, he'd pick the Ph.D. every time. Sure, he said, he'd bet on the sculptor's being more physically talented; but he'd bet on the Ph.D.'s being less "flaky." And in the end that matters more. Skill, surgeons believe, can be taught; tenacity cannot. It's an odd approach to recruitment, but it continues all the way up the ranks, even in top surgery departments. They start with minions with no experience in surgery, spend years training them, and then take most of their faculty from these same homegrown ranks.

And it works. There have now been many studies of elite performers—concert violinists, chess grand masters, professional ice skaters, mathematicians, and so forth—and the biggest difference researchers find between them and lesser performers is the amount of deliberate practice they've accumulated. Indeed, the most important talent may be the talent for practice itself. K. Anders Ericsson, a cognitive psychologist and an expert on performance, notes that the most important role that innate factors play may be in a person's *willingness* to engage in sustained training. He has found, for example, that top performers dislike practicing just as much as others do. (That's why, for example, athletes and musicians usually quit practicing when they retire.) But, more than others, they have the will to keep at it anyway.

I wasn't sure I did. What good was it, I wondered, to keep doing central lines when I wasn't coming close to hitting them? If I had a clear idea of what I was doing wrong, then maybe I'd have something to focus on. But I didn't. Everyone, of course, had suggestions. Go in with the bevel of the needle up. No, go in with the bevel down. Put a bend in the middle of the needle. No, curve the needle. For a while, I tried to avoid doing another line. Soon enough, however, a new case arose.

The circumstances were miserable. It was late in the day, and I'd had to work through the previous night. The patient weighed more than three hundred pounds. He couldn't tolerate lying flat because the weight of his chest and abdomen made it hard for him to breathe. Yet he had a badly infected wound, needed intravenous antibiotics, and no one could find veins in his arms for a peripheral IV. I had little hope of succeeding. But a resident does what he is told, and I was told to try the line.

I went to his room. He looked scared and said he didn't think he'd last more than a minute on his back. But he said he understood the situation and was willing to make his best effort. He and I decided that he'd be left sitting propped up in bed until the last possible minute. We'd see how far we got after that.

I went through my preparations: checking his blood counts from the lab, putting out the kit, placing the towel roll, and so on. I swabbed and draped his chest while he was still sitting up. S., the chief resident, was watching me this time, and when everything was ready I had her tip him back, an oxygen mask on his face. His flesh rolled up his chest like a wave. I couldn't find his clavicle with my fingertips to line up the right point of entry. And already he was looking short of breath, his face red. I gave S. a "Do you want to take over?" look. Keep going, she signaled. I made a rough guess about where the right spot was, numbed it with lidocaine, and pushed the big needle in. For a second, I thought it wouldn't be long enough to reach through, but then I felt the tip slip underneath his clavicle. I pushed a little deeper and drew back on the syringe. Unbelievably, it filled with blood. I was in. I concentrated on anchoring the needle firmly in place, not moving it a millimeter as I pulled the syringe off and threaded the guide wire in. The wire fed in smoothly. The patient was struggling hard for air now. We sat him up and let him catch his breath. And then, laying him down one more time, I got the entry dilated and slid the central line in. "Nice job" was all S. said, and then she left.

I still have no idea what I did differently that day. But from then on my lines went in. That's the funny thing about practice. For days and days, you make out only the fragments of what to do. And then one day you've got the thing whole. Conscious learning becomes unconscious knowledge, and you cannot say precisely how.

I have now put in more than a hundred central lines. I am by no means infallible. Certainly, I have had my fair share of complications. I punctured a patient's lung, for example—the right lung of a chief of surgery from another hospital, no less—and, given the odds, I'm sure such things will happen again. I still have the occasional case that should go easily but doesn't, no matter what I do. (We have a term for this. "How'd it go?" a colleague asks. "It was a total flog," I reply. I don't have to say anything more.)

But other times everything unfolds effortlessly. You take the needle. You stick the chest. You feel the needle travel—a distinct glide through the fat, a slight catch in the dense muscle, then the subtle pop through the vein wall—and you're in. At such moments, it is more than easy; it is beautiful.

Surgical training is the recapitulation of this process—floundering followed by fragments followed by knowledge and, occasionally, a moment of elegance—over and over again, for ever harder tasks with ever greater risks. At first, you work on the basics: how to glove and gown, how to drape patients, how to hold the knife, how to tie a square knot in a length of silk suture (not to mention how to dictate, work the computers, order drugs). But then the tasks become more daunting: how to cut through skin, handle the electrocautery, open the breast, tie off a bleeder, excise a tumor, close up a wound. At the end of six months, I had done lines, lumpectomies, appendectomies, skin grafts, hernia repairs, and mastectomies. At the end of a year, I was doing limb amputations, hemorrhoidectomies, and laparoscopic gallbladder operations. At the end of two years, I was beginning to do tracheotomies, small-bowel operations, and leg-artery bypasses.

I am in my seventh year of training, of which three years have been spent doing research. Only now has a simple slice through skin begun to seem like the mere start of a case. These days, I'm trying to learn how to fix an abdominal aortic aneurysm, remove a pancreatic cancer, open blocked carotid arteries. I am, I have found, neither gifted nor maladroit. With practice and more practice, I get the hang of it.

Doctors find it hard to talk about this with patients. The moral burden of practicing on people is always with us, but for the most part it is unspoken. Before each operation, I go over to the holding area in my scrubs and introduce myself to the patient. I do it the same way every time. "Hello, I'm Dr. Gawande. I'm one of the surgical residents, and I'll be assisting your surgeon." That is pretty much all I say on the subject. I extend my hand and smile. I ask the patient if everything is going OK so far. We chat. I answer questions. Very occasionally, patients are taken aback. "No resident is doing my surgery," they say. I try to be reassuring. "Not to worry—I just assist," I say. "The attending surgeon is always in charge."

None of this is exactly a lie. The attending *is* in charge, and a resident knows better than to forget that. Consider the operation I did recently to remove a seventy-five-year-old woman's colon cancer. The attending stood across from me from the start. And it was he, not I, who decided where to cut, how to position the opened abdomen, how to isolate the cancer, and how much colon to take.

Yet I'm the one who held the knife. I'm the one who stood on the operator's side of the table, and it was raised to my six-foot-plus height. I was there to help, yes, but I was there to practice, too. This was clear when it came time to reconnect the colon. There are two ways of putting the ends together—handsewing and stapling. Stapling is swifter and easier, but the attending suggested I handsew the ends—not because it was better for the patient but because I had had much less experience doing it. When it's performed correctly, the results are similar, but he needed to watch me like a hawk. My stitching was slow and imprecise. At one point, he caught me putting the stitches too far apart and made me go back and put extras in between so the connection would not leak. At another point, he found I wasn't taking deep enough bites of tissue with the needle to ensure a strong closure. "Turn your wrist more," he told me. "Like this?" I asked. "Uh, sort of," he said.

In medicine, there has long been a conflict between the imperative to give patients the best possible care and the need to provide novices with experience. Residencies attempt to mitigate potential harm through supervision and graduated responsibility. And there is reason to think that patients actually benefit from teaching. Studies commonly find that teaching hospitals have better outcomes than non-teaching hospitals. Residents may be amateurs, but having them around checking on patients, asking questions, and keeping faculty on their toes seems to help. But there is still

no avoiding those first few unsteady times a young physician tries to put in a central line, remove a breast cancer, or
sew together two segments of colon. No matter how many
protections are in place, on average these cases go less well
with the novice than with someone experienced.

Doctors have no illusions about this. When an attending
physician brings a sick family member in for surgery, people
at the hospital think twice about letting trainees participate.
Even when the attending insists that they participate as
usual, the residents scrubbing in know that it will be far
from a teaching case. And if a central line must be put in, a
first-timer is certainly not going to do it. Conversely, the
ward services and clinics where residents have the most
responsibility are populated by the poor, the uninsured, the
drunk, and the demented. Residents have few opportunities
nowadays to operate independently, without the attending
docs scrubbed in, but when we do—as we must before graduating and going out to operate on our own—it is generally
with these, the humblest of patients.

And this is the uncomfortable truth about teaching. By
traditional ethics and public insistence (not to mention court
rulings), a patient's right to the best care possible must
trump the objective of training novices. We want perfection
without practice. Yet everyone is harmed if no one is trained
for the future. So learning is hidden, behind drapes and
anesthesia and the elisions of language. And the dilemma
doesn't apply just to residents, physicians in training. The
process of learning goes on longer than most people know.

I grew up in the small Appalachian town of Athens, Ohio,
where my parents are both doctors. My mother is a pediatrician and my father is a urologist. Long ago, my mother chose

to practice part time, which she could afford to do because my father's practice became so busy and successful. He has now been at it for more than twenty-five years, and his office is cluttered with the evidence of this. There is an overflowing wall of medical files, gifts from patients displayed everywhere (books, paintings, ceramics with biblical sayings, hand-painted paperweights, blown glass, carved boxes, a figurine of a boy who, when you pull down his pants, pees on you), and, in an acrylic case behind his oak desk, a few dozen of the thousands of kidney stones he has removed.

Only now, as I get glimpses of the end of my training, have I begun to think hard about my father's success. For most of my residency, I thought of surgery as a more or less fixed body of knowledge and skill which is acquired in training and perfected in practice. There was, I thought, a smooth, upward-sloping arc of proficiency at some rarefied set of tasks (for me, taking out gallbladders, colon cancers, bullets, and appendixes; for him, taking out kidney stones, testicular cancers, and swollen prostates). The arc would peak at, say, ten or fifteen years, plateau for a long time, and perhaps tail off a little in the final five years before retirement. The reality, however, turns out to be far messier. You do get good at certain things, my father tells me, but no sooner do you master something than you find that what you know is outmoded. New technologies and operations emerge to supplant the old, and the learning curve starts all over again. "Three-quarters of what I do today I never learned in residency," he says. On his own, fifty miles from his nearest colleague—let alone a doctor who could tell him anything like "You need to turn your wrist more"—he has had to learn to put in penile prostheses, to perform microsurgery, to reverse vasectomies, to do nerve-sparing prostatectomies, to implant artificial urinary sphincters. He's had to learn to use shock-wave lithotripters, electrohydraulic lithotripters, and laser lithotripters (all instruments for breaking up kidney stones); to deploy Double J ureteral stents and Silicone Figure Four Coil stents and Retro-Inject Multi-Length stents (don't even ask); and to maneuver fiber-optic ureteroscopes. All these technologies and techniques were introduced after he finished training. Some of the procedures built on skills he already had. Many did not.

This is the experience that all surgeons have. The pace of medical innovation has been unceasing, and surgeons have no choice but to give the new thing a try. To fail to adopt new techniques would mean denying patients meaningful medical advances. Yet the perils of the learning curve are inescapable—no less in practice than in residency.

For the established surgeon, inevitably, the opportunities for learning are far less structured than for a resident. When an important new device or procedure comes along, as happens every year, surgeons start by taking a course about it—typically a day or two of lectures by some surgical grandees with a few film clips and step-by-step handouts. You take home a video to watch. Perhaps you pay a visit to observe a colleague perform the operation—my father often goes up to the Cleveland Clinic for this. But there's not much by way of hands-on training. Unlike a resident, a visitor cannot scrub in on cases, and opportunities to practice on animals or cadavers are few and far between. (Britain, being Britain, actually bans surgeons from practicing on animals.) When the pulse-dye laser came out, the manufacturer set up a lab in Columbus where urologists from the area could gain experience. But when my father went there the main experience provided was destroying kidney stones in test tubes filled with a urinelike liquid and trying to penetrate the shell of an egg without hitting the membrane underneath. My surgery department recently bought a robotic surgery device—a staggeringly sophisticated nine-hundred-and-eighty-thousand-dollar robot, with three arms, two wrists, and a camera, all millimeters in diameter, which, controlled from a console, allows a surgeon to do almost any operation with no hand tremor and with only tiny incisions. A team of two surgeons and two nurses flew out to the manufacturer's headquarters, in Mountain View, California, for a full day of training on the machine. And they did get to practice on a pig and on a human cadaver. (The company apparently buys the cadavers from the city of San Francisco.) But even this was hardly thorough training. They learned enough to grasp the principles of using the robot, to start getting a feel for using it, and to understand how to plan an operation. That was about it. Sooner or later, you just have to go home and give the thing a try on someone.

Patients do eventually benefit—often enormously—but the first few patients may not, and may even be harmed. Consider the experience reported by the pediatric cardiac-surgery unit of the renowned Great Ormond Street Hospital, in London, as detailed in the *British Medical Journal* last April. The doctors described their results from 325 consecutive operations between 1978 and 1998 on babies with a severe heart defect known as transposition of the great arteries. Such children are born with their heart's outflow vessels transposed: the aorta emerges from the right side of the heart instead of the left and the artery to the lungs emerges from the left instead of the right. As a result, blood coming in is pumped right back out to the body instead of first to the lungs, where it can be oxygenated. The babies died blue, fatigued, never knowing what it was to get enough breath. For years, it wasn't technically feasible to switch the vessels to their proper positions. Instead, surgeons did something known as the Senning procedure: they created a passage inside the heart to let blood from the lungs cross backward to the right heart. The Senning procedure allowed children to live into adulthood. The weaker right heart, however, cannot sustain the body's entire blood flow as long as the left. Eventually, these patients' hearts failed, and although most survived to adulthood, few lived to old age.

By the 1980s, a series of technological advances made it possible to do a switch operation safely, and this became the favored procedure. In 1986, the Great Ormond Street surgeons made the changeover themselves, and their report shows that it was unquestionably an improvement. The annual death rate after a successful switch procedure was less than a quarter that of the Senning, resulting in a life expectancy of sixty-three years instead of forty-seven. But the price of learning to do it was appalling. In their first seventy switch operations, the doctors had a 25 percent surgical death rate, compared with just 6 percent with the Senning procedure. Eighteen babies died, more than twice the number during the entire Senning era. Only with time did they master it: in their next hundred switch operations, five babies died.

As patients, we want both expertise and progress; we don't want to acknowledge that these are contradictory desires. In the words of one British public report, "There should be no learning curve as far as patient safety is concerned." But this is entirely wishful thinking.

Recently, a group of Harvard Business School researchers who have made a specialty of studying learning curves in industry decided to examine learning curves among surgeons instead of in semiconductor manufacture or airplane construction, or any of the usual fields their colleagues examine. They followed eighteen cardiac surgeons and their teams as they took on the new technique of minimally invasive cardiac surgery. This study, I was surprised to discover, is the first of its kind. Learning is ubiquitous in medicine, and yet no one had ever compared how well different teams actually do it.

The new heart operation—in which new technologies allow a surgeon to operate through a small incision between ribs instead of splitting the chest open down the middle—proved substantially more difficult than the conventional one. Because the incision is too small to admit the usual tubes and clamps for rerouting blood to the heart-bypass machine, surgeons had to learn a trickier method, which involved balloons and catheters placed through groin vessels. And the nurses, anesthesiologists, and perfusionists all had new roles to master. As you'd expect, everyone experienced a substantial learning curve. Whereas a fully proficient team takes three to six hours for such an operation, these teams took on average three times as long for their early cases. The researchers could not track complication rates in detail, but it would be foolish to imagine that they were not affected.

What's more, the researchers found striking disparities in the speed with which different teams learned. All teams came from highly respected institutions with experience in adopting innovations and received the same three-day training session. Yet, in the course of fifty cases, some teams managed to halve their operating time while others improved hardly at all. Practice, it turned out, did not necessarily make perfect. The crucial variable was *how* the surgeons and their teams practiced.

Richard Bohmer, the only physician among the Harvard researchers, made several visits to observe one of the quickest-learning teams and one of the slowest, and he was startled by the contrast. The surgeon on the fast-learning team was actually quite inexperienced compared with the one on the slow-learning team. But he made sure to pick team members with whom he had worked well before and to keep them together through the first fifteen cases before allowing any new members. He had the team go through a dry run before the first case, then deliberately scheduled six operations in the first week, so little would be forgotten in between. He convened the team before each case to discuss it in detail and afterward to debrief. He made sure results were tracked carefully. And Bohmer noticed that the surgeon was not the stereotypical Napoleon with a knife. Unbidden, he told Bohmer, "The surgeon needs to be willing to allow himself to become a partner [with the rest of the team] so he can accept input." At the other hospital, by contrast, the surgeon chose his operating team almost randomly and did not keep it together. In the first seven cases, the team had different members every time, which is to say that it was no team at all. And the surgeon had no prebriefings, no debriefings, no tracking of ongoing results.

The Harvard Business School study offered some hopeful news. We can do things that have a dramatic effect on our rate of improvement—like being more deliberate about how we train, and about tracking progress, whether with students and residents or with senior surgeons and nurses. But the study's other implications are less reassuring. No matter how accomplished, surgeons trying something new got worse before they got better, and the learning curve proved longer, and was affected by a far more complicated range of factors, than anyone had realized.

This, I suspect, is the reason for the physician's dodge: the "I just assist" rap; the "We have a new procedure for this that you are perfect for" speech; the "You need a central line" without the "I am still learning how to do this." Sometimes we do feel obliged to admit when we're doing something for the first time, but even then we tend to quote the published complication rates of experienced surgeons. Do we ever tell patients that, because we are still new at something, their risks will inevitably be higher, and that they'd likely do better with doctors who are more experienced? Do we ever say that we need them to agree to it anyway? I've never seen it. Given the stakes, who in his right mind would agree to be practiced upon?

Many dispute this presumption. "Look, most people understand what it is to be a doctor," a health policy expert insisted, when I visited him in his office not long ago. "We have to stop lying to our patients. Can people take on choices for societal benefit?" He paused and then answered his question. "Yes," he said firmly.

It would certainly be a graceful and happy solution. We'd ask patients—honestly, openly—and they'd say yes. Hard to imagine, though. I noticed on the expert's desk a picture of his child, born just a few months before, and a completely unfair question popped into my mind. "So did you let the resident deliver?" I asked.

There was silence for a moment. "No," he admitted. "We didn't even allow residents in the room."

One reason I doubt whether we could sustain a system of medical training that depended on people saying "Yes, you can practice on me" is that I myself have said no. When my eldest child, Walker, was eleven days old, he suddenly went into congestive heart failure from what proved to be a severe cardiac defect. His aorta was not transposed, but a long segment of it had failed to grow at all. My wife and I were beside ourselves with fear—his kidneys and liver began failing, too—but he made it to surgery, the repair was a success, and although his recovery was erratic, after two and a half weeks he was ready to come home.

We were by no means in the clear, however. He was born a healthy six pounds plus but now, a month old, he weighed only five, and would need strict monitoring to ensure that he gained weight. He was on two cardiac medications from which he would have to be weaned. And in the longer term, the doctors warned us, his repair would prove inadequate. As Walker grew, his aorta would require either dilation with a balloon or replacement by surgery. They could not say precisely when and how many such procedures would be necessary over the years. A pediatric cardiologist would have to follow him closely and decide.

Walker was about to be discharged, and we had not indicated who that cardiologist would be. In the hospital, he had been cared for by a full team of cardiologists, ranging from fellows in specialty training to attendings who had practiced for decades. The day before we took Walker home, one of the young fellows approached me, offering his card and suggesting a time to bring Walker to see him. Of those on the team, he had put in the most time caring for Walker. He saw Walker when we brought him in inexplicably short of breath, made the diagnosis, got Walker the drugs that stabilized him, coordinated with the surgeons, and came to see us twice a day to answer our questions. Moreover, I knew, this was how fellows always got their patients. Most families don't know the subtle gradations among players, and after a team has saved their child's life they take whatever appointment they're handed.

But I knew the differences. "I'm afraid we're thinking of seeing Dr. Newburger," I said. She was the hospital's associate cardiologist-in-chief, and a published expert on conditions like Walker's. The young physician looked crestfallen. It was nothing against him, I said. She just had more experience, that was all.

"You know, there is always an attending backing me up," he said. I shook my head.

I know this was not fair. My son had an unusual problem. The fellow needed the experience. As a resident, I of all people should have understood this. But I was not torn about the decision. This was my child. Given a choice, I will always choose the best care I can for him. How can anybody be expected to do otherwise? Certainly, the future of medicine should not rely on it.

In a sense, then, the physician's dodge is inevitable. Learning must be stolen, taken as a kind of bodily eminent domain. And it was, during Walker's stay—on many occasions, now that I think back on it. A resident intubated him. A surgical trainee scrubbed in for his operation. The cardiology fellow put in one of his central lines. If I had the option to have someone more experienced, I would have taken it. But this was simply how the system worked—no such choices were offered—and so I went along.

The advantage of this coldhearted machinery is not merely that it gets the learning done. If learning is necessary but causes harm, then above all it ought to apply to everyone alike. Given a choice, people wriggle out, and such choices are not offered equally. They belong to the connected and the knowledgeable, to insiders over outsiders, to the doctor's child but not the truck driver's. If everyone cannot have a choice, maybe it is better if no one can.

It is 2:00 p.m. I am in the intensive-care unit. A nurse tells me Mr. G.'s central line has clotted off. Mr. G. has been in the hospital for more than a month now. He is in his late sixties, from South Boston, emaciated, exhausted, holding on by a thread—or a line, to be precise. He has several holes in his small bowel, and the bilious contents leak out onto his skin through two small reddened openings in the concavity of his abdomen. His only chance is to be fed by vein and wait for these fistulae to heal. He needs a new central line.

I could do it, I suppose. I am the experienced one now. But experience brings a new role: I am expected to teach the procedure instead. "See one, do one, teach one," the saying goes, and it is only half in jest.

There is a junior resident on the service. She has done only one or two lines before. I tell her about Mr. G. I ask her if she is free to do a new line. She misinterprets this as a question. She says she still has patients to see and a case coming up later. Could I do the line? I tell her no. She is unable to hide a grimace. She is burdened, as I was burdened, and perhaps frightened, as I was frightened.

She begins to focus when I make her talk through the steps—a kind of dry run, I figure. She hits nearly all the steps, but forgets about checking the labs and about Mr. G.'s nasty allergy to heparin, which is in the flush for the line. I make sure she registers this, then tell her to get set up and page me.

I am still adjusting to this role. It is painful enough taking responsibility for one's own failures. Being handmaiden to another's is something else entirely. It occurs to me that I could have broken open a kit and had her do an actual dry run. Then again maybe I can't. The kits must cost a couple of hundred dollars each. I'll have to find out for next time.

Half an hour later, I get the page. The patient is draped. The resident is in her gown and gloves. She tells me that she has saline to flush the line with and that his labs are fine.

"Have you got the towel roll?" I ask.

She forgot the towel roll. I roll up a towel and slip it beneath Mr. G.'s back. I ask him if he's all right. He nods. After all he's been through, there is only resignation in his eyes.

The junior resident picks out a spot for the stick. The patient is hauntingly thin. I see every rib and fear that the resident will puncture his lung. She injects the numbing medication. Then she puts the big needle in, and the angle looks all wrong. I motion for her to reposition. This only makes her more uncertain. She pushes in deeper and I know she does not have it. She draws back on the syringe: no blood. She takes out the needle and tries again. And again the angle looks wrong. This time, Mr. G. feels the jab and jerks up in pain. I hold his arm. She gives him more numbing medication. It is all I can do not to take over. But she cannot learn without doing, I tell myself. I decide to let her have one more try.

The Infernal Chorus

ROBERT JAY LIFTON

On March 30, 1979, after having lived in Munich for almost seven months, I hosted a small party to say goodbye to a few of my friends. At the gathering I told one of them that I was "tired of interviewing Nazis," and that I was not surprised but nonetheless troubled that not one of them had made a genuine moral confrontation of past behavior.

That night I had a dream in which I was part of a male singing group, a version of a barbershop quartet, and we were about to sing something. But I knew that it was no ordinary group, that it was an "infernal chorus," and was vaguely aware, even in the dream, that infernal meant the underworld, hell, death. I woke up with the phrase "infernal chorus" reverberating in my head, and quickly associated it with the voices of Nazi doctors. My interviews with them had made me part of the chorus, and I was expressing my discomfort at "singing" with such a group. I was feeling a strong need to sing my own song, detach myself from the infernal chorus, and have my say about it.

In one sense I was simply following my general pattern of returning from work in the field to the solitude of my American study to give structure and meaning to that work. What was different this time was my convoluted relationship with the country from which I was returning. I never forgot that, during their twelve-year Nazi binge, German leaders and large numbers of German people wanted to murder me along with all other Jews. At the same time I was aware of how much I valued the bonds I formed with individual Germans, many of whom were remarkable in their intelligence, sensibility, and dedication. Our shared confrontation of grotesque historical details infused our colleagueship with special intensity and our friendships with special affection.

I think of many warm dinners with Iring and Elisabeth Fetscher in Frankfurt. Iring, a political philosopher and leading German intellectual voice, contributed to my work at every level. He even appeared on a panel with me on Nazi doctors and, himself an authority on Marxism, defended my research against a Marxist critic who faulted me for a psychological rather than an economic emphasis. Elisabeth took loving care of me when I developed a gastrointestinal condition while staying at their home. Their son Sebastian, a physician who spent time in America, visited us at Wellfleet and became one of the German translators of my book. And their other son Justus, a literary scholar, hosted us in Berlin and taught me much about German generational struggles in connection with the Nazi era. My wife, BJ, and I had a memorable experience with the Fetschers as a family (two of their three adult children were present) in viewing together in early 1979 an episode of the German version of the American television series *Holocaust*. The original film was in many ways flawed, and had a mixed reception in the United States, but for many Germans it was an important historical event, evoking in a number of viewers confessional memories and expressions of guilt in connection with behavior at the time. The Fetschers had insisted that we rush through dinner to be able to see the film. We all watched it in silence, though Elisabeth sobbed during a portion depicting the killing of Jews, and no one had much to say afterward. But we knew we had experienced a moment of communion in confronting together what Germans had done to Jews.

Nazi Doctors on My Desk

Yet even when leaving Nazi doctors behind in Germany, I was far from rid of them. Facing my records of them, my thousands of pages of interviews and notes, was just as difficult as talking to them. I remember a revealing moment soon after my return when I walked into my Wellfleet study, perhaps my favorite room in the world, to find myself completely devoid of the pleasure I usually experienced when entering it. Great piles of folders on my large desk made me feel completely alone with Nazi doctors. Until then I had been somewhat protected from taking in fully what they had been part of and what they had done by the very activity required for arranging and carrying out the interviews. Now I had no such protection, and knew that I had no choice but to permit Nazi doctors to dominate my imagination so that I could interpret their behavior and compose what I had to say about them. Only by writing that book could I get them out of my study.

At the same time I was struggling psychologically with my whole German experience. As I wrote to Iring Fetscher, "BJ and I are still very much in transition spiritually. . . . I find that all kinds of things are working on me internally." Some of what was working on me came out in two kinds of dreams I was then having. One category was that of transition dreams involving European locales and activities as well as amorphous journeys. In one such dream I was in London uneasily seeking out two destinations: an open-air sports facility that somehow resembled a Nazi camp, and an obscure "massage parlor." I noted the next day the dream's unpleasant juxtaposition of "athletics, sex, and the Nazi death camps." In these transition dreams I could not seem to settle into, or even locate, a destination. I felt well described by A. R. Ammons in his poem "Return," where he speaks of coming "a long way/without arriving" and of climbing a peak but finding "no foothold/higher than the ground."

The second category I called death dreams, and they were more eerie and disturbing. They involved people who had died but appeared as sometimes vigorous phantoms: my father, my mother, Robert Vas, Les Farber. Those dreams reminded me in turn of two earlier dreams: In one of them a friend notified me that my obituary had appeared in *The New York Times* and I checked and found it to be there. And in another dream, I observed someone spreading ashes, only to realize that the ashes being spread were my own. My psyche had long been accumulating macabre death imagery, and that process was greatly intensified by my exposure to Nazi doctors. I was surviving my travels among the dead, but not easily. Heinrich Böll's observation that "the artist carries his death within him like a good priest his breviary" extends, I believe, to the psychological witness of mass killing and dying.

I also seemed to require life-giving antidotes, some of which were expressed in other dreams I had that I related to healing. At about that time I had an additional dream that I still remember with some pleasure. It consisted solely of two neatly printed words, "Vatican grapes," surrounded by a vine of actual purple grapes to form an attractive tableau. It was clear to me even during the dream that the grapes were (as I wrote the next day) "associated with healing." While I have never been a particular fan of the Vatican, I thought of

Pope John XXIII, the appealing ecumenical figure who, from 1958 to 1963, sought to heal the Catholic Church in its relationship to the world. I thought also of the healing encounters I had personally experienced with such Catholic figures as the Berrigans, Joe O'Rourke, and Bishop Barker. But the dream also seemed humorous, and when I told BJ about it we bantered about producing a healing elixir called "Vatican Grapes" that would make us rich, speculating on whether we would need permission from the pope for a patent, and on considering a brand of "Jewish Grapes" as well. And in my note I had a little fun with associations to "grapes"—"sour grapes, Grapes of Wrath, food, wine, Dionysus, orgies, languid sexual feeling." Maybe I was desperate for antidotes.

In working on the book and on articles and talks along the way, I was concerned—and not without cause, as it turned out—about how such emotionally freighted material would be received. When I spoke at medical schools and hospitals, physicians mostly raised thoughtful questions about potential American transgressions, such as giving lethal injections in carrying out executions, involvement in military violence as in Vietnam, or being socialized by their medical institutions to various forms of callous behavior. Psychiatrists and psychoanalysts tended to be fascinated by the psychological motivations of Nazi doctors and interested in my personal struggles over the course of the work. But there were notable exceptions, for instance doctors who were angered by suggestions of parallels of any kind with what American doctors did, insisting that Nazi behavior be seen as unique and unrelated to that of anyone else.

There were also more extreme reactions. I still have an image in my mind of the prominent psychoanalyst who stormed up to the podium after my presentation and screamed into the microphone: "I don't give a damn about what's in the mind of a Nazi doctor! I don't want to know what he's thinking or feeling!"—with a vehemence that temporarily disrupted the professional meeting. I responded by insisting on the importance of grasping motivations of Nazi doctors in order to combat the kind of behavior they represented and the kind of system they were part of. I was troubled by the incident because it threatened the rationale of my entire study. Together with a supportive colleague, I wrote a letter to the sponsoring psychoanalytic group, insisting on our profession's obligation to probe the most disturbing questions, in accordance with the Enlightenment principle "Dare to know!" I still believe strongly in that principle, but must confess a certain retrospective sympathy for the protesting psychoanalyst's simple outrage. I have frequently felt the same way myself.

My struggles in writing the book had to do not only with the extremity of the subject matter, but as always with structure, in this case with the kind of structure that could best encompass the full dimensions of what I had observed. Now the mosaic had to include the broad Nazi biomedical vision, leading from sterilization to "euthanasia" to the death camps, as well as detailed exploration of the psychology of Auschwitz as an institution and of individual Nazi doctors who served it. In the last section of the volume, I extended the mosaic to include a systematic grid of what I took to be the overall psychological steps of any genocide. I found getting this book written especially demanding, and the help of an astute editor crucial. The editor, to my good fortune, was my friend Jane Isay, who had edited several of my earlier books, had an unusual grasp of my work in general, and offered her counsel during trips to Wellfleet as well as in New York City. Were it not for her, those Nazi doctors might still be sitting on my desk.

More of the Infernal Chorus

The Nazi Doctors had more prepublication exposure than any of my other books. Largely through the strong interest of Abe Rosenthal, executive editor and dictator-in-chief of *The New York Times,* two chapters were adapted into full-length *Times Magazine* articles, one on Mengele and the other on the "euthanasia" program. My friendship with Abe was long-standing and ambivalent: I admired his early critical reporting in the late fifties from Poland and in the sixties from Japan (including sympathetic writings on Hiroshima survivors), where we were able to spend some time together. Unfortunately, he was to turn into a petulant reactionary, partly through backlash to the sixties, and came to alienate almost everyone around him. When he died in 2006 I had not seen him for almost two decades, but I am still grateful for the intensity with which he embraced my work on Nazi doctors and contributed to the launching of my book.

The Nazi Doctors received an anguished front-page Sunday *New York Times* review by Bruno Bettelheim, a psychoanalyst who was himself a survivor of Nazi camps but a controversial figure because of attacks on other survivors, including those of death camps, for alleged compromises they had made with Nazi jailers. In a similar vein he questioned my efforts to understand the motivations of Nazi doctors and ended his review with the enigmatic acknowledgment: "For this reason I may not have been able to do full justice to this book."

But I have come to realize that such a review, and a number of others as well, were a kind of extension of that "infernal chorus" from which I had to struggle to extricate myself. The moral insanity of the Nazi doctors reverberated in ways that could evoke a reaction that was itself caught up in the madness. My book was an attempt to expose that grotesque chorus, and in writing it I had to suppress my own rage, including sentiments not too different from those of Bettelheim. It would seem that any immersion into the world of Nazi doctors runs the risk of entering into that infernal chorus. Fortunately, the great majority of reviewers stepped back from it sufficiently to open themselves to what I was trying to do. I was especially pleased by the response of Neal Ascherson, the British journalist and historian, in *The New York Review of Books* because he affirmed what I most wished the book to convey: a way of grasping how Nazi doctors could do what they did, and a new and useful approach to the Nazi movement that was both psychological and historical. I had no idea that the work would have later relevance for American doctors and their collusion in torture during the Iraq War era.

I began this section by saying there were moments when I could not believe I'd done any such work on Nazi doctors; the same was true about writing a book about them. My own work, I now realize, was a constant struggle to connect with the "separate planet" mentioned by both Nazi doctors and inmates, to make Auschwitz real to others and to myself. While I knew there had to be a cost, I have never been much inclined to examine that cost, partly because of my awareness that whatever the study did to me pales before the suffering of actual victims and survivors. But I think there was also involved a certain research macho pride in viewing myself as one who can deal with such painful matters.

BJ has always said that the Nazis turned my hair gray—it had been almost black—and if so, there was probably involved an element of survivors' despair concerning the human potential for such behavior. But the pain is inseparable from a sense that the work is a culmination of my life as a researcher. When the book was completed and published, I found myself saying that I could now better accept dying because something elemental in me had been realized. A friend once asked me whether, knowing what I know now, would I make the same decision to do the study—to which I replied that I would anticipate and share the dread of people close to me but would very likely go ahead with the project.

fiction

We Are Nighttime Travelers

ETHAN CANIN

Where are we going? Where, I might write, is this path leading us? Francine is asleep and I am standing downstairs in
the kitchen with the door closed and the light on and a stack
of mostly blank paper on the counter in front of me. My
dentures are in a glass by the sink. I can clean them with a
tablet that bubbles in the water, and although they were
clean already I just cleaned them again because the bubbles
are agreeable and I thought their effervescence might excite
me to write. But words fail me.

This is a love story. However, its roots are tangled and
involve a good bit of my life, and when I recall my life my
mood turns sour and I am reminded that no man makes
truly proper use of his time. We are blind and small-minded.
We are dumb as snails and as frightened, full of vanity and
misinformed about the importance of things. I'm an average
man, without great deeds except maybe one, and that has
been to love my wife.

I have been more or less faithful to Francine since I married her. There has been one transgression—leaning up
against a closet wall with a red-haired purchasing agent at a
sales meeting once in Minneapolis twenty years ago; but she
was buying auto upholstery and I was selling it and in the
eyes of judgment this may bear a key weight. Since then,
though, I have ambled on this narrow path of life bound to

a woman. This is a triumph and a regret. In our current state of affairs it is a regret because in life a man is either on the uphill or on the downhill, and if he isn't procreating he is on the downhill. It is a steep downhill indeed. These days I am tumbling, falling headlong among the scrub oaks and boulders, tearing knees and abrading all bony parts of the body. I have given myself to gravity.

Francine and I are married now forty-six years, and I would be a bamboozler to say that I have loved her for any more than half of these. Let us say that for the last year I haven't; let us say this for the last ten, even. Time has made torments of our small differences and tolerance of our passions. This is our state of affairs. Now I stand by myself in our kitchen in the middle of the night; now I lead a secret life. We wake at different hours now, sleep in different corners of the bed. We like different foods and different music, keep our clothing in different drawers, and if it can be said that either of us has aspirations, I believe that they are to a different bliss. Also, she is healthy and I am ill. And as for conversation—our house is silent as the bone yard.

Last week we did talk. "Frank," she said one evening at the table, "there is something I must tell you."

The New York game was on the radio, snow was falling outside, and the pot of tea she had brewed was steaming on the table between us. Her medicine and my medicine were in little paper cups at our places.

"Frank," she said, jiggling her cup, "what I must tell you is that someone was around the house last night."

I tilted my pills onto my hand. "Around the house?"

"Someone was at the window."

On my palm the pills were white, blue, beige, pink: Lasix, Diabinese, Slow-K, Lopressor. "What do you mean?"

She rolled her pills onto the tablecloth and fidgeted with

them, made them into a line, then into a circle, then into a line again. I don't know her medicine so well. She's healthy, except for little things. "I mean," she said, "there was someone in the yard last night."

"How do you know?"

"Frank, will you really, please?"

"I'm asking you how you know."

"I heard him," she said. She looked down. "I was sitting in the front room and I heard him outside the window."

"You heard him?"

"Yes."

"The front window?"

She got up and went to the sink. This is a trick of hers. At a distance I can't see her face.

"The front window is ten feet off the ground," I said.

"What I know is that there was a man out there last night, right outside the glass." She walked out of the kitchen.

"Let's check," I called after her. I walked into the living room, and when I got there she was looking out the window.

"What is it?"

She was peering out at an angle. All I could see was snow, blue-white.

"Footprints."

I built the house we live in with my two hands. That was forty-nine years ago, when, in my foolishness and crude want of learning, everything I didn't know seemed like a promise. I learned to build a house and then I built one. There are copper fixtures on the pipes, sanded edges on the struts and queen posts. Now, a half-century later, the floors are flat as a billiard table but the man who laid them needs two hands to pick up a woodscrew. This is the diabetes. My feet are gone also. I look down at them and see two black shapes when I walk, things I can't feel. Black clubs. No connection with the ground. If I didn't look, I could go to sleep with my shoes on.

Life takes its toll, and soon the body gives up completely. But it gives up the parts first. This sugar in the blood: God says to me: "Frank Manlius—codger, man of prevarication and half-truth—I shall take your life from you, as from all men. But first—" But first! Clouds in the eyeball, a heart that makes noise, feet cold as uncooked roast. And Francine, beauty that she was—now I see not much more than the dark line of her brow and the intersections of her body; mouth and nose, neck and shoulders. Her smells have changed over the years so that I don't know what's her own anymore and what's powder.

We have two children, but they're gone now too, with children of their own. We have a house, some furniture, small savings to speak of. How Francine spends her day I don't know. This is the sad truth, my confession. I am gone past nightfall. She wakes early with me and is awake when I return, but beyond this I know almost nothing of her life.

I spend my days at the aquarium. I've told Francine something else, of course, that I'm part of a volunteer service of retired men, that we spend our days setting young businesses afoot: "Immigrants," I told her early on, "newcomers to the land." I said it was difficult work. In the evenings I could invent stories, but I don't, and Francine doesn't ask.

I am home by nine or ten. Ticket stubs from the aquarium fill my coat pocket. Most of the day I watch the big sea

animals—porpoises, sharks, a manatee—turn their saltwa-
ter loops. I come late morning and move a chair up close.
They are wanting to eat then. Their bodies skim the cool
glass, full of strange magnifications. I think, if it is possible,
that they are beginning to know me: this man—hunched at
the shoulder, cataractic of eye, breathing through water
himself—this man who sits and watches. I do not pity
them. At lunchtime I buy coffee and sit in one of the hotel
lobbies or in the cafeteria next door, and I read poems.
Browning, Whitman, Eliot. This is my secret. It is night
when I return home. Francine is at the table, four feet across
from my seat, the width of two drop-leaves. Our medicine is
in cups. There have been three presidents since I held her in
my arms.

The cafeteria moves the men along, old or young, who come
to get away from the cold. A half-hour for a cup, they let me
sit. Then the manager is at my table. He is nothing but
polite. I buy a pastry then, something small. He knows
me—I have seen him nearly every day for months now—
and by his slight limp I know he is a man of mercy. But business is business.

"What are you reading?" he asks me as he wipes the
table with a wet cloth. He touches the saltshaker, nudges the
napkins in their holder. I know what this means.

"I'll take a cranberry roll," I say. He flicks the cloth and
turns back to the counter.

This is what:

Shall I say, I have gone at dusk through narrow streets
And watched the smoke that rises from the pipes
Of lonely men in shirt-sleeves, leaning out of windows?

Through the magnifier glass the words come forward, huge, two by two. With spectacles, two by two. With spectacles everything is twice enlarged. Still, though, I am slow to read it. In a half-hour I am finished, could not read more, even if I bought another roll. The boy at the register greets me, smiles when I reach him. "What are you reading today?" he asks, counting out the change.

The books themselves are small and fit in the inside pockets of my coat. I put one in front of each breast, then walk back to see the fish some more. These are the fish I know: the gafftopsail pompano, sixgill shark, the starry flounder with its upturned eyes, queerly migrated. He rests half-submerged in sand. His scales are platey and flat-hued. Of everything upward he is wary, of the silvery seabass and the bluefin tuna that pass above him in the region of the light and open water. For a life he lies on the bottom of the tank. I look at him. His eyes are dull. They are ugly and an aberration. Above us the bony fishes wheel at the tank's corners. "Platichthys stellatus," I say to him. The caudal fin stirs. Sand moves and resettles, and I see the black and yellow stripes. "Flatfish," I whisper, "we are, you and I, observers of this life."

"A man on our lawn," I say a few nights later in bed.
   "Not just that."
   I breathe in, breathe out, look up at the ceiling.
   "What else?"
   "When you were out last night he came back."
   "He came back?"
   "Yes."
   "What did he do?"
   "Looked in at me."

Later, in the early night, when the lights of cars are still passing and the walked dogs still jingle their collar chains out front, I get up quickly from bed and step into the hall. I move fast because this is still possible in short bursts and with concentration. The bed sinks once, then rises. I am on the landing and then downstairs without Francine waking. I stay close to the staircase joists.

In the kitchen I take out my almost-blank sheets and set them on the counter. I write standing up because I want to take more than an animal's pose. For me this is futile, but I stand anyway. The page will be blank when I finish. This I know. The dreams I compose are the dreams of others, remembered bits of verse. Songs of greater men than I. In months I have written few more than a hundred words. The pages are stacked, sheets of different sizes.

If I could

one says,

It has never seemed

says another. I stand and shift them in and out. They are mostly blank, sheets from months of nights. But this doesn't bother me. What I have is patience.

Francine knows nothing of the poetry. She's a simple girl, toast and butter. I myself am hardly the man for it: forty years selling (anything—steel piping, heater elements, dried bananas). Didn't read a book except one on sales. Think victory, the book said. Think *sale*. It's a young man's bag of apples, though; young men in pants that nip at the waist.

Ten years ago I left the Buick in the company lot and walked home, dye in my hair, cotton rectangles in the shoulders of my coat. Francine was in the house that afternoon also, the way she is now. When I retired we bought a camper and went on a trip. A traveling salesman retires, so he goes on a trip. Forty miles out of town the folly appeared to me, big as a balloon. To Francine, too. "Frank," she said in the middle of a bend, a prophet turning to me, the camper pushing sixty and rocking in the wind, trucks to our left and right, big as trains—"Frank," she said, "these roads must be familiar to you."

So we sold the camper at a loss and a man who'd spent forty years at highway speed looked around for something to do before he died. The first poem I read was in a book on a table in a waiting room. My eyeglasses made half-sense of things.

> *THESE*
> *are the desolate, dark weeks.*

I read,

> *when nature in its barrenness*
> *equals the stupidity of man.*

Gloom, I thought, and nothing more, but when I reread the words, and suddenly there I was, hunched and wheezing, bald as a trout, and tears were in my eye. I don't know where they came from.

* * *

In the morning an officer visits. He has muscles, mustache, skin red from the cold. He leans against the door frame.

"Can you describe him?" he says.

"It's always dark," says Francine.

"Anything about him?"

"I'm an old woman. I can see that he wears glasses."

"What kind of glasses?"

"Black."

"Dark glasses?"

"Black glasses."

"At a particular time?"

"Always when Frank is away."

"Your husband has never been here when he's come?"

"Never."

"I see." He looks at me. This look can mean several things, perhaps that he thinks Francine is imagining. "But never at a particular time?"

"No."

"Well," he says. Outside on the porch his partner is stamping his feet. "Well," he says again. "We'll have a look." He turns, replaces his cap, heads out to the snowy steps. The door closes. I hear him say something outside.

"Last night—," Francine says. She speaks in the dark. "Last night I heard him on the side of the house."

We are in bed. Outside, on the sill, snow has been building since morning.

"You heard the wind."

"Frank." She sits up, switches on the lamp, tilts her head toward the window. Through a ceiling and two walls I can hear the ticking of our kitchen clock.

"I heard him climbing," she says. She has wrapped her arms about her own waist. "He was on the house. I heard him. He went up the drainpipe." She shivers as she says this.

"There was no wind. He went up the drainpipe and then I heard him on the porch roof."

"Houses make noise."

"I heard him. There's gravel there."

I imagine the sounds, amplified by hollow walls, rubber heels on timber. I don't say anything. There is an arm's length between us, cold sheet, a space uncrossed since I can remember.

"I have made the mistake in my life of not being interested in enough people," she says then. "If I'd been interested in more people, I wouldn't be alone now."

"Nobody's alone," I say.

"I mean that if I'd made more of an effort with people, I would have friends now. I would know the postman and the Giffords and the Kohlers, and we'd be together in this, all of us. We'd sit in each other's living rooms on rainy days and talk about the children. Instead we've kept to ourselves. Now I'm alone."

"You're not alone," I say.

"Yes, I am." She turns the light off and we are in the dark again. "You're alone, too."

My health has gotten worse. It's slow to set in at this age, not the violent shaking grip of death; instead—a slow leak, nothing more. A bicycle tire: rimless, thready, worn treadles already and now losing its fatness. A war of attrition. The tall camels of the spirit steering for the desert. One morning I realized I hadn't been warm in a year.

And there are other things that go, too. For instance, I recall with certainty that it was on the twenty-third of April, 1945, that despite German counteroffensives in the Ardennes, Eisenhower's men reached the Elbe; but I cannot remember whether I have visited the savings and loan this week. Also, I am unable to produce the name of my neighbor, though I greeted him yesterday in the street. And take, for example, this: I am at a loss to explain whole decades of my life. We have children and photographs, and there is an understanding between Francine and me that bears the weight of nothing less than a half a century, but when I gather my memories they seem to fill no more than an hour. Where has my life gone?

It has gone partway to shoddy accumulations. In my wallet are credit cards, a license ten years expired, twenty-three dollars in cash. There is a photograph but it depresses me to look at it, and a poem, half-copied and folded into the billfold. The leather is pocked and has taken on the curve of my thigh. The poem is from Walt Whitman. I copy only what I need.

But of all things to do last, poetry is a barren choice. Deciphering other men's riddles while the world is full of procreation and war. A man should go out swinging an axe. Instead, I shall go out in a coffee shop.

But how can any man leave this world with honor? Despite anything he does, it grows corrupt around him. It fills with locks and sirens. A man walks into a store now and the microwaves announce his entry; when he leaves, they make electronic peeks into his coat pockets, his trousers. Who doesn't feel like a thief? I see a policeman now, any policeman, and I feel a fright. And the things I've done wrong in my life haven't been crimes. Crimes of the heart perhaps, but nothing against the state. My soul may turn black but I can wear white trousers at any meeting of men. Have I loved my wife? At one time, yes—in rages and torrents. I've been covered by the pimples of ecstasy and have rooted in the mud of despair; and I've lived for months, for whole years now, as mindless of Francine as a tree of its mosses.

And this is what kills us, this mindlessness. We sit across the tablecloth now with our medicines between us, little balls and oblongs. We sit, sit. This has become our view of each other, a tableboard apart. We sit.

"Again?" I say.

"Last night."

We are at the table. Francine is making a twisting motion with her fingers. She coughs, brushes her cheek with her forearm, stands suddenly so that the table bumps and my medicines move in the cup.

"Francine," I say.

The half-light of dawn is showing me things outside the window: silhouettes, our maple, the eaves of our neighbor's garage. Francine moves and stands against the glass, hugging her shoulders.

"You're not telling me something," I say.

She sits and makes her pills into a circle again, then into a line. Then she is crying.

I come around the table, but she gets up before I reach her and leaves the kitchen. I stand there. In a moment I hear a drawer open in the living room. She moves things around, then shuts it again. "Sit down," she says. When she returns she sits at the other side of the table. She puts two folded sheets of paper onto the table. "I wasn't hiding them," she says.

"What weren't you hiding?"

"These," she says. "He leaves them.

"They say he loves me."

"Francine."

"They're inside the windows in the morning." She picks one up, unfolds it. Then she reads:

"Ah, I remember well (and how can I
But evermore remember well) when first . . ."

She pauses, squint-eyed, working her lips. It is a pause of only faint understanding. Then she continues.

"Our flame began, when scarce we knew what was
The flame we felt. . . ."

When she finishes she refolds the paper precisely. "That's it," she says. "That's one of them."

At the aquarium I sit, circled by glass and, behind it, the senseless eyes of fish. I have never written a word of my own poetry but can recite the verse of others. This is the culmination of a life. *Coryphaena hippurus,* says the plaque on the dolphin's tank, words more beautiful than any of my own. The dolphin circles, circles, approaches with alarming speed, but takes no notice of, if he even sees, my hands. I wave them in front of his tank. What must he think has become of the sea? He turns and his slippery proboscis nudges the glass. I am every part sore from life.

Ah, silver shrine, here will I take my rest
After so many hours of toil and quest,
A famished pilgrim,—saved by miracle.

There is nothing noble for either of us here, nothing between us, and no miracles. I am better off drinking cof-

fee. Any fluid refills the blood. The counter boy knows me
and later at the café he pours the cup, most of a dollar's
worth. Refills are free but my heart hurts no different from
a bone, bruised or cracked. This amazes.

Francine is amazed by other things. She is mystified,
thrown beam ends by the romance. She reads me the poems
now at breakfast, one by one. I sit. I roll my pills. "Another
came last night," she says, and I see her eyebrows rise.
"Another this morning." She reads them as if every word is
a surprise. Her tongue touches teeth, shows between lips.
These lips are dry. She reads:

> "Kiss me as if you made believe
> You were not sure, this eve,
> How my face, your flower, had pursed
> Its petals up."

That night she shows me the windowsill, second story,
rimmed with snow, where she finds the poems. We open the
glass. We lean into the air. There is ice below us, sheets of it
on the trellis, needles hanging from the drainwork.

"Where do you find them?"

"Outside," she says. "Folded, on the lip."

"In the morning?"

"Always in the morning."

"The police should know about this."

"What will they be able to do?"

I step away from the sill. She leans out again, surveying
her lands, which are the yard's-width spit of crusted ice
along our neighbor's chain-link and the three maples out
front, now lost their leaves. She peers as if she expects this
man to appear. An icy wind comes inside. "Think," she
says. "Think. He could come from anywhere."

* * *

One night in February, a month after this began, she asks
me to stay awake and stand guard until the morning. It is
almost spring. The earth has reappeared in patches. During
the day, at the borders of yards and driveways, I see glimpses
of brown—though I know I could be mistaken. I come home
early that night, before dusk, and when darkness falls I
move a chair by the window downstairs. I draw apart the
outer curtain and raise the shade. Francine brings me a pot
of tea. She turns out the light and pauses next to me, and as
she does, her hand on the chair's backbrace, I am so struck
by the proximity of elements—of the night, of the teapot's
heat, of the sounds of water outside—that I consider speaking. I want to ask her what has become of us, what has made
our breathed air so sorry now, and loveless. But the timing
is wrong and in a moment she turns and climbs the stairs. I
look out into the night. Later, I hear the closet shut, then
our bed creak.

There is nothing to see outside, nothing to hear. This I
know. I let hours pass. Behind the window I imagine fish
moving down to greet me: broomtail grouper, surfperch,
sturgeon with their prehistoric rows of scutes. It is almost
possible to see them. The night is full of shapes and bits of
light. In it the moon rises, losing the colors of the horizon,
so that by early morning it is high and pale. Frost has made
a ring around it.

A ringed moon above, and I am thinking back on things.
What have I regretted in my life? Plenty of things, mistakes
enough to fill the car showroom, then a good deal of the
back lot. I've been a man of gains and losses. What gains?

My marriage, certainly, though it has been no knee-buckling windfall but more like a split decision in the end, a stock risen a few points since bought. I've certainly enjoyed certain things about the world, too. These are things gone over and over again by the writers and probably enjoyed by everybody who ever lived. Most of them involve air. Early morning air, air after a rainstorm, air through a car window. Sometimes I think the cerebrum is wasted and all we really need is the lower brain, which I've been told is what makes the lungs breathe and the heart beat and what lets us smell pleasant things. What about the poetry? That's another split decision, maybe going the other way if I really made a tally. It's made me melancholy in old age, sad when if I'd stuck with motor homes and the national league standings I don't think I would have been rooting around in regret and doubt at this point. Nothing wrong with sadness, but this is not the real thing—not the death of a child but the feelings of a college student reading *Don Quixote* on a warm afternoon before going out to the lake.

Now, with Francine upstairs, I wait for a night prowler. He will not appear. This I know, but the window glass is ill-blown and makes moving shadows anyway, shapes that change in the wind's rattle. I look out and despite myself am afraid.

Before me, the night unrolls. Now the tree leaves turn yellow in moonshine. By two or three, Francine sleeps, but I get up anyway and change into my coat and hat. The books weigh against my chest. I don gloves, scarf, galoshes. Then I climb the stairs and go into our bedroom, where she is sleeping. On the far side of the bed I see her white hair and beneath the blankets the uneven heave of her chest. I watch the bedcovers rise. She is probably dreaming at this moment. Though we have shared this bed for most of a lifetime I cannot guess what her dreams are about. I step next to her and touch the sheets where they lie across her neck.

"Wake up," I whisper. I touch her cheek, and her eyes open. I know this though I cannot really see them, just the darkness of their sockets.

"Is he there?"

"No."

"Then what's the matter?"

"Nothing's the matter," I say. "But I'd like to go for a walk."

"You've been outside," she says. "You saw him, didn't you?"

"I've been at the window."

"Did you see him?"

"No. There's no one there."

"Then why do you want to walk?" In a moment she is sitting aside the bed, her feet in slippers. "We don't ever walk," she says.

I am warm in all my clothing. "I know we don't," I answer. I turn my arms out, open my hands toward her. "But I would like to. I would like to walk in air that is so new and cold."

She peers up at me. "I haven't been drinking," I say. I bend at the waist, and though my head spins, I lean forward enough so that the effect is of a bow. "Will you come with me?" I whisper. "Will you be queen of this crystal night?" I recover from my bow, and when I look up again she has risen from the bed, and in another moment she has dressed herself in her wool robe and is walking ahead of me to the stairs.

Outside, the ice is treacherous. Snow has begun to fall and our galoshes squeak and slide, but we stay on the ploughed walkway long enough to leave our block and enter a part of the neighborhood where I have never been. Ice hangs from the lamps. We pass unfamiliar houses and unfamiliar trees, street signs I have never seen, and as we walk the night begins to change. It is becoming liquor. The snow is banked on either side of the walk, ploughed into hillocks at the corners. My hands are warming from the exertion. They are the hands of a younger man now, someone else's fingers in my gloves. They tingle. We take ten minutes to cover a block but as we move through this neighborhood my ardor mounts. A car approaches and I wave, a boatman's salute, because here we are together on these rare and empty seas. We are nighttime travelers. He flashes his headlamps as he passes, and this fills me to the gullet with celebration and bravery. The night sings to us. I am Bluebeard now, Lindbergh, Genghis Khan.

No, I am not.

I am an old man. My blood is dark from hypoxia, my breaths singsong from disease. It is only the frozen night that is splendid. In it we walk, stepping slowly, bent forward. We take steps the length of table forks. Francine holds my elbow.

I have mean secrets and small dreams, no plans greater than where to buy groceries and what rhymes to read next, and by the time we reach our porch again my foolishness has subsided. My knees and elbows ache. They ache with a mortal ache, tired flesh, the cartilage gone sandy with time. I don't have the heart for dreams. We undress in the hallway, ice in the ends of our hair, our coats stiff from cold. Francine turns down the thermostat. Then we go upstairs and she gets into her side of the bed and I get into mine.

It is dark. We lie there for some time, and then, before dawn, I know she is asleep. It is cold in our bedroom. As I listen to her breathing I know my life is coming to an end. I cannot warm myself. What I would like to tell my wife is this:

> *What the*
> *imagination*
> *seizes*
> *as beauty must be truth. What holds you*
> *to what you see of me is*
> *that grasp alone.*

But I do not say anything. Instead I roll in the bed, reach across, and touch her, and because she is surprised she turns to me.

When I kiss her the lips are dry, cracking against mine, unfamiliar as the ocean floor. But then the lips give. They part. I am inside her mouth, and there, still, hidden from the world, as if ruin had forgotten a part, it is wet—Lord! I have the feeling of a miracle. Her tongue comes forward. I do not know myself then, what man I am, who I lie with in embrace. I can barely remember her beauty. She touches my chest and I bite lightly on her lip, spread moisture to her cheek and then kiss there. She makes something like a sigh. "Frank," she says. "Frank." We are lost now in seas and deserts. My hand finds her fingers and grips them, bone and tendon, fragile things.

Dog 1, Dog 2

NICK EARLS

You are unsure of all of this, but maybe that's just you.

Ever since the Dean lined you up for The Influence, If Any, Of Maternal Low-Dose Piroxicam On The Development Of The Sublingual Fat Pad In Fetal Marmosets as your doctoral thesis, you have realized that the world progresses in particularly small steps, some of them (some of the biggest) backward and a great many sideways in screaming lunatic tangents, arms flapping, lips slathering, eyes bulging with the glee of infinitesimal discovery. Such, you feel, is your work with, for, and on behalf of the marmosets. They didn't thank you. Their eyes bulged only with a feral, shuffling ignorance. Ignorance of your intent, ignorance of their antenatal exposure to piroxicam and its implications (if any), ignorance even of their own sublingual fat pads. Science barely thanked you either. It gave you your doctorate, one paper, one lecture, and a one-way ticket to more of this.

So now you are here, at Kranfield Pharmaceuticals, with perhaps your only progress the fact that you no longer work under the insipid gaze of marmosets. This is not an insipid lab. It is under the control of a man called Robert who is far from insipid. He is, in fact, a complete shit.

He seems to ooze when he moves, and he has great difficulty controlling flatulence. At times, when you are updating him about your work, his cheeks redden, his eyes bulge (though not with the innocence of marmosets), and he stares a good distance away, maneuvering uncomfortably on his lab stool. It is as though he is carefully digesting what you are telling him and, realizing its worthlessness, he is about to shit it in front of you. You go out of your way to make your reports hard, nuggety, pointed, just to put pain on his face as he purges himself of your cleverness.

All of this is part of the unspoken collective consciousness of the lab. That which has been spoken allows a disgruntled worker to refer to a bad day as one that would really give you the Roberts.

The man is a shit, and though it's not just your problem you feel it more keenly than most, as the only other person in the lab with a doctorate.

The main thrust of your present work involves dogs. Someone at Kranfield has taken the familiar piroxicam molecule (a fine drug and a great earner, but, regrettably, someone else's), fiddled with a side-chain, and slapped a patent on the end result. You have to prove that it's safe for humans, or, at least, unlikely to be downright dangerous. You do this with dogs, and in increasingly large doses.

Now, dogs aren't cheap, so you can't do it with thousands. Unfortunately, you have a small enough number to name them, chat to them, invent personalities for them with the help of the technicians. Dog One becomes Rowan, after your large and lazy brother-in-law; Dog Two becomes AB, following his excellence in specific physical tests, the fact that he's an all-round good bloke with the respect of the whole team, and a general feeling that he would be more than willing to stand up to the most venomous eight-foot West Indian fast bowler, and with a straight bat too. And so it goes.

You are clearly bored with the work, but perhaps you

should have thought this naming business through. You should have learned all the necessary lessons about scientific detachment around the time you were snipping the tongues from newborn marmosets. But revulsion soon gave way to statistics, writing, proofreading, revising, waiting, waiting, waiting. And then word from the Dean that the examiners were giving the thumbs-up.

And the Dean had a contact at Kranfield Pharmaceuticals, and here you are.

And out comes the new piroxicam derivative, so where are the marmosets? But this time it's Labradors. And they wag their tails when you feed them something munchy after giving them forty times the recommended human dose of the drug. You know you have to do this, you know that people can't be the first. But what about Rowan, AB, Wozza, Nataly, and the rest? All so happy to see you in the morning.

You exercise them vigorously twice a day to maximize opportunities for wear and tear. Periodically, you X-ray their knees. Eventually, you will look at the tissues of their knee joints under a microscope, administering various stains to assess progression of disease, or degree of cartilage preservation.

One night, in a dream, you set them free. All of them. You see them bounding through the night with knees glowing from numerous X-rays. Wafting silently into the distance like a blissful cloud of fireflies. And you are alone. There is an unpleasant smell, and a fart cracks the night like a walnut, and Robert is beside you. Questioning you. Oozing again. You depress his tongue with a spatula and pump in several liters of the drug, which then sets like concrete. His face goes red and he looks over your shoulder, grunting with some discomfort. In the enormous effort to shit he splits in two, the last thing to collapse into the rubble his bewildered puffed-up face.

But you are unlikely to do the world this much good in your entire life. You are a known killer of marmosets, about to move on to animals that actually like you.

On the bus into the city, you would tell people, explain yourself. Explain that you are doing it for them. But striking up a conversation about marmosets, your marmosets, or even your Labradors, would be as welcome as telling them how much better your life has been since you met Jesus. And offering them some helpful literature. A woman once did this to you on a bus, and then she hit you for a donation. So now if anyone says hi you just look straight ahead. No one says hi.

You change buses in town. In the second bus, too, no one says hi. People talk only to people they already know, so you have no chance to unburden yourself, or to make any religious purchases. The bus works its way through the commuter traffic, and the passengers, who all appear to be students, are talking about their distaste for eight o'clock lectures and their plans to seek extensions for assignments. And you want to tell them about the real world. You want to tell them that when they were born someone might have cut their tongues out to check the fat pads. But no one did, and they don't know how lucky they are.

But one or two of them do look a little like marmosets. And you imagine that the bus is rocking along a lonely dirt road late at night and you are a prisoner of the marmosets. And they look at you with those eyes again. They turn and they look at you over the seats and they say nothing. They show you their empty mouths, they show you they have no tongues, and they never take their eyes off you. Dozens of them. You find an old pamphlet pushed down next to the seat. You pull it out as though it might distract them, and you say, Jesus anyone?

At this moment, you realize you are holding an empty barbecue-chip packet between the heads of the two students sitting in front of you. They decline politely, as if it is clear to them you are disturbed, but not dangerous. They move up to the front of the bus to tell their friends about the madman who just offered them Cheezels from an empty barbecue-chip packet. There is considerable laughter at your expense. Students are like that. Despite the embarrassment, you are not glad when your stop arrives.

At morning tea, you crunch through a plateful of the hard, wheaty biscuits of which you have grown fond, and real life doesn't hold too many answers.

And Robert doesn't make things any easier. He's becoming even more territorial, even more protective of what he's doing. Less willing to let you into his office, even though access to the computer is essential to your work. He sits in the corner scratching himself, grumbling under his breath, making smells. And you are glad to enter your data and leave.

You tell him you should wait a good time before killing the dogs, or the work will have little value. You're not going soft are you? he says. You wouldn't catch me going soft. And he laughs a hoarse laugh and he bares his teeth. He is a compendium of unpleasant habits, and they're only getting worse.

You return to the exercise yard to run the dogs. They're pleased to see you. They jump up to you, paw you like drunk friends, sniff your pockets for biscuits, start raising their own doubts with you, like, why are we here? Does all this, this life thing, have any meaning? And you tell them they have been chosen. For what? they ask. Not unreasonably. Well, this is basically a holiday camp, a sort of Club Med thing, lots of team activities, you tell them. And they've won a prize, each of them, and the prize is that they get to spend a very long holiday here. Three meals a day and plenty of exercise and fun. And you tell them you have to return to work now, and you go inside.

You notice a calendar and realize it's a long time since you took your worm tablets. You pop two from a blister pack, and you mix them in with a bowl of appetizing soft food and devour it enthusiastically. But of course you then spit the tablets back into the bowl, and get fairly pissed off with yourself. You've never been good with tablets.

You mix up the next few days' worth of the drug, at a higher dose now for some of the dogs. And you aren't happy about this, but it tastes OK.

The next day is someone's birthday, so you all bring along lunch. One of the others has brought soy chicken wings, a known favorite of Robert's. He watches you all as he pulls the flesh from the bones, watches you all 'cause he knows you want it too. And then he crunches the bones, but in his haste starts spluttering, coughing, turning purplish. Some dickhead hits him in the back and he coughs up the bone fragment, turns pinkish again, drools quietly with relief.

The man is a shit, and you'd like nothing more than to see him whitening by the roadside, crumbling into powder, slowly dissipated by the wind.

You have a bit of a doze after lunch, and when you wake you give yourself a good going over with a stiff brush. And you feel all shiny and clean, even though the others don't notice.

And Rowan's not looking well. He makes it clear he's

feeling distinctly queasy, and he wonders if it's what you're pumping into him. It could be just the birthday lunch, you tell him. Labradors can eat too much too quickly and not feel the best. But he was feeling sick before lunch. He didn't eat any lunch. Let's see how it goes, you say, there's a bit of it around and in fact I'm not feeling so well myself. And you feel your nose, just to show you're monitoring things. Rowan really isn't looking well, and he goes for a lie down.

It's hard to concentrate on your work after this. After you haven't even bothered to come up with a good lie for him. Surely he's worth more than this, you tell yourself. And you really don't feel well and you want to go home for the afternoon. You'd tell Robert about it, but he's pacing up and down in his office, basically grumbling and scratching himself, and he's obviously anxious about something. He's tugging at his uncomfortable shirt and you notice how old and worn the collar looks. And he scratches under his arms and he scratches his flanks and he scratches behind his ears.

So you just go home.

The next morning is one of those mornings when you wake up feeling as though you've copped a bait, and you're off your breakfast and you head for work with no enthusiasm whatsoever.

And Rowan's cage is empty. Big, happy Rowan. One of the others tells you he started throwing up blood during the night, and no one came when they called for help, and it didn't last long. And Robert's somewhere with his knee joints, and he's not very happy. This could bugger up the whole thing. It's not the result the company wants at all. Great knees maybe, but not a great drug if the patient's dead.

And Robert will have to hold someone responsible for

this. And even though you stuck strictly to protocol, you know it will be you.

You are told he wants to see you at five, when all the others have gone. And at five, all the others go, and it's no use curling up in the corner on your blanket whimpering.

You hear his feet on the lino, his heavy panting breathing, smell that Robert smell. He snarls at you with contempt when he sees you cowering there, growls cruelly. And you know he's offering you only one way out.

You back across the room and he follows you, checking your ineffectual moves to escape, growling ever more menacingly. And you back into the empty Dog One cage and he shuts the wire door. He prowls around the cage, obviously tense, and you sit in the basket looking pathetic and making inadvertent whining noises. He comes right up to the wire, shows you all his teeth, backs off again. His smell is suffocating. Before he leaves, to make his position clear, he squats at the cage door, his face goes bulge-eyed and distant, and he drops a large shit to the lino floor.

He laughs at you with heavy, wet breathing, and he clatters off down the hallway.

And as you wait for the morning, a morning meaning a heavy, pasty dose of the piroxicam derivative, a bowl of something crunchy, and more exercise than you're used to, Robert bounds through the night, baying at the moon in anger and triumph.

He stops, to concentrate hard on another shit, and as he lets it go, feels that calm feeling of letting it go, he is clubbed from behind by the proprietor of a nearby Chinese restaurant who is finding the going tough in these times of recession, and needs to come by his Mongolian lamb through other than conventional means.

He drags the body onto the back of his ute, making sure not to step in the shit, which over the following several months whitens by the roadside, crumbles into powder, and is slowly dissipated by the wind.

And in his absence, and with a number of the dogs developing side effects, the new molecule is abandoned, the experiment erased, and you end up with a nice family in the suburbs. And in summer they take you to their holiday house at the coast, where you run on the beach for hours. And at sunset you jump and snap, but only playfully, at the fireflies.

The Duty to Die Cheaply

PETER GOLDSWORTHY

"If there is a doctor on board the aircraft, please identify yourself by pressing the attendant call-button. I repeat . . ."

Heads craned all along the cabin: Who needed a doctor? And where? Dr. Philip Shaw—3A, Business Class—craned his head for one reason only: in the hope that a better Samaritan might reach up for the call-button first. How long could he decently wait? He was out of practice—epidemiology left no time for the sharpening of clinical skills. Worse, he had been drinking. The announcement ended abruptly, the river Vivaldi flowed again through his headphones—Light Classics, Channel 4, Inflight Entertainment. He rapidly drained his third complimentary scotch and glanced at his watch: the second hand slipped a cog, then another. Worst-case scenario: cardiac arrest, four minutes to brain death. Could he afford to wait even one more second? He had waited no more than five when an attendant leaned in over him, clutching a passenger manifest.

"Doctor Shaw? Doctor Philip Shaw."

He lifted his hand and pressed the call-button above his head, absurdly, automatically. The red call-light glowed, fingering him publicly. You got me. His neighbors in Business—charcoal suits and silvered heads mostly—turned and examined him; he tried not to make eye contact.

"I'll come quietly," he said.

The cabin attendant was all whispered, suppressed agitation. "Doctor, one of the passengers is rather unwell. If you could follow me, please . . ."

He rose immediately and followed her back into Economy, running a gauntlet of stares that was definitely more judgmental than up front. 25C, aisle seat. The victim—male, overweight, gray-pepper beard—appeared terrifyingly still. The two adjacent seats had been emptied; the ejected passengers stood in the entrance to the rear galley, trying not to watch, yet of course watching. The purser—a painstakingly groomed older woman who had earlier fetched Philip his scotches—was bent over the victim, pressing a mask to his face. A young male attendant was wrestling with the valve of an oxygen cylinder. The cylinder distracted Philip momentarily; it seemed for some reason to have been designed according to aerodynamic principles, a tiny version of the aircraft itself, clean-lined and slender, lacking only wings.

"This is Mr. Brice, Doctor," the purser said.

The victim was long past introductions. He was also past oxygen. Kneeling in the aisle, Philip checked the neck pulses—absent. A clammy sweat covered the brow—heart attack, almost certainly. The pupils were fixed and dilated.

Various emotions washed through him, among them a definite gust of relief. The late Mr. Brice had been dead for some time, well before the intercom's first summons.

He reached across and gently twisted shut the oxygen valve. His eyes met the purser's; she held his gaze.

"His neighbor thought he was asleep," she said, simply.

Philip stepped back into the aisle, made superfluous by death. The routines of the cabin crew which followed seemed well practiced: the seat was reclined, the seat belt lengthened and buckled about the victim's big body, the two flaccid hands placed carefully in his lap. Lastly, the head, face, and upper torso were draped with a cabin blanket.

The woman in the row immediately in front of the dead man—a young, harried mother, traveling with two small girls—turned, disbelieving. "You're going to *leave* him there?"

The purser's tone was smooth and soothing. "Space is at a premium, madam. There is the galley, but—you will understand—health regulations forbid . . ."

Busy with her daughters, the woman may or may not have heard the reply. "I said face the *front,* Simone!"

Philip had a jokey, slightly drunk suggestion: "Is there room on the flight deck?"

The purser affected not to hear. He was tempted to try again—some variation on flying on autopilot—but the words would not quite come together. Those quickfire scotches on an empty stomach were beginning to fuzz his brain. He needed a fourth.

"Well, if there's nothing else I can do."

It seemed there was. The purser plucked at his sleeve, subtly detaining him.

"Doctor, I realize it's an imposition, but the flight is fully booked, and it would be a great help if you would agree to sit with the, ah, patient."

Philip stared into her face, surprised for the first time that day, though not unpleasantly. The unexpected had become a rare commodity in recent years; he was learning to savor it.

"You want me to sit with a dead man?"

"Just for the remaining minutes of the flight."

He glanced at his watch. "That would be . . . ninety remaining minutes? Give or take."

He felt loosened by the whisky, even a little reckless, but the purser remained unfazed.

"Doctor, please. We could hardly expect someone, ah, inexperienced, to sit with the deceased."

Philip glanced about the cabin. Fait accompli: the two displaced passengers had vanished forward, a Business Class upgrade, at his expense.

He squeezed in past the fat, shrouded body—no simple matter—and eased himself into the window seat.

"There might be an undertaker on board," he said to the purser, lightheartedly. "Perhaps you could make an announcement."

"Please, Doctor. If you could fasten your seat belt."

The purser vanished, but the attendant who had earlier summoned him from Business Class was now leaning in, a younger woman wearing a fixed, cheery smile, her hair tugged back into the tightest of plaits.

"Can I get you anything, Doctor?"

"Flyspray?"

Her smile remained cheery, as if tethered by the same tight drawstrings that bound back her hair.

"Sorry," he excused himself. "But if you don't laugh, you cry."

The woman in 24C turned her head again.

"Excuse me, but *I'd* like to change seats. I really don't think my children can be expected to sit here in front of that poor man."

"I'll see what I can do," the attendant promised.

"I'll have a scotch," Philip got in before she left. "And my valise, please."

"Of course, Doctor."

"In the overhead locker. 3A."

More whisky arrived, a jug of water, ice, and a whispered apology to the concerned-mother-of-two, "There is simply no other seating available, madam."

Philip unscrewed the mini-bottle—Johnny Walker, Black Label, nothing special—and drank it neat. The first shot burnt his mouth pleasantly, the next smoked down into his chest, relaxing him deeply, and somehow warming his heart en route. His cold heart, according to some. He smiled over the intervening shroud at a young woman seated across the aisle; she glanced away.

"Another?" he waved the little empty bottle, trying to catch the attendant's eye, but now she was pushing the lunch trolley, working backward, row by row, offering meal trays. As she neared the rear of the cabin there appeared to be fewer takers.

"Would you care for some lunch, madam?"

"Hardly!" the woman in 24C said.

"And the children?"

"They're not hungry, either."

"But, *Mum*—"

"Hush. We'll have something at Grandma's."

"But I'm *hungry*."

The trolley rolled on.

"I don't suppose you will be wanting any lunch, Doctor?"

He looked up into that determined smile. "In fact, yes," he said. "Please. And some wine."

She handed him a shrink-wrapped plastic tray, reaching across high above the body. He handed it back.

"Business Class," he reminded her.

Her smile remained cryptic, but there was something in the eyes: definite distaste. Was it the company he was keeping? He smiled to himself, amused by his own private joke.

"And might I have another scotch while I wait?"

She passed down another Johnny Walker, topped his jug of water and plastic cup of ice, then wheeled her trolley past. The purser arrived shortly with the menu card, and—reaching across the shrouded body with difficulty—set a starched linen napkin on his lap. The card seemed difficult to read for some reason, hard to bring into focus, but he chose the fish—barramundi—and the sauvignon blanc, and when the food arrived ate hungrily enough, the flow of digestive juices released, as always, by alcohol. Pots of coffee were offered about as he tucked into the crème caramel, the passengers in the vicinity of the body once again refusing to partake.

He ordered a cognac after the meal had been cleared, and reclined his chair fully, feeling weirdly, weightlessly happy, a lighter-than-air machine himself, floating inside this larger flying machine. He unsealed the headphones in the seat pocket, slipped them on, and tuned to Channel 4. Albinoni this time, or some such tranquilizer. He tried to listen, but the earpieces were uncomfortable, hard little Economy Class rubbers, lacking foam padding, and he soon removed them.

A small girl's face began to appear by increments above the top of the seat in front, blonde fringe first, wide possum eyes, thimble nose. He passed her the chocolate after-dinner mint from his tray, pressing a finger to his lips, "Ssh."

Her face ducked out of sight, only to reappear, by slow degrees, a few seconds later, her mouth wearing an uneven coat of chocolate lipstick.

"Boo!" he said.

She giggled, her head ducked down again, and again slowly reemerged. He played the game twice more before tiring of it. His own children—teenagers now—had long cured him of the joys of repetition. The fourth time the little face poked above the seat, he reached across to his dead neighbor and flipped aside the corner of blanket that veiled the face.

The child's wide eyes widened even further; she vanished as if jerked down into her seat. This time, she failed to reappear; he could hear a mother's whispered scolding.

He looked sideways at Mr. Brice, unmasked. With his own chair reclined, he found himself at eye level with the corpse, with just the raised middle seat between them. He reached over and reclined that seat also, affording a better view. The dead man's face, pale and cooling, had relaxed, freed from any emotional expression. Liberated, was the word that sprang to Philip's mind. The eyes had the dull, milky look of death. Only the beard—soft, springy, gray-flecked—still looked alive, which of course it was. And no doubt growing, slowly.

"So," Philip said aloud, slurring the sibilants a little, "what if I need a piss?"

No answer. The pressure of the seat belt against his full bladder was growing; he hoped he could hold on. He replaced the shroud, drained his cognac, and tried to attract the young attendant's eye. Was she avoiding him? She had clearly formed a wrong impression; he felt an urge to defend himself. I *was* going to answer the summons, he wanted to tell her. I was merely waiting for someone better qualified. He banged the empty glass down on the tray, making the point. My practice hasn't been made of patients for a long time, he explained—if only to himself—but made of paper. A house of index cards. And electronic bytes. Electronic bricks: cost-benefit statistics, survival-rate data. Quality-of-life indices. Moreover, in the past I have *always* answered the call. I fly a lot; there have been a lot of calls. And not only in planes. The theater, the movies . . .

Why can't it be someone else's turn? he wanted to

demand of her. Because even when I *do* report for duty, other people fuck it up. Including your colleagues, Miss Tight Lips. Let me tell you of the time I was flying Adelaide–Frankfurt, and the dread call came. Congestive heart failure, an old dear drowning in her own foaming fluids . . .

He closed his eyes, and was thrown back, giddily, to that day, that flight. He had pressed an oxygen mask to the woman's face; still she had choked. The remedy had been obvious: she had needed to lose a liter or two of fluid from those lungs. In that overbooked jumbo, at least one passenger would be very likely carrying diuretics, he had reasoned. Yet the cabin crew had refused to broadcast a plea for "water tablets." Against company policy, Doctor. We cannot risk being sued for incorrectly prescribed drugs.

He had suggested—with some venom—that the only alternative was to fly at a lower altitude. And so the huge ship, as much zeppelin as jet plane, had lumberingly descended, on medical advice, to three thousand feet, and remained there, at enormous cost in fuel consumption, for the rest of the flight, and the drowning woman had survived.

His reward? *Danke schön, Herr Doktor,* and a bottle of wine. Not even an upgrade out of cattle class. Wood class, in German.

He opened his eyes. A bottle of wine might at least help him get over his current assignment: babysitting the dead. He turned back to his traveling companion. The first corpse he had seen, years before, came back to him through the thickening fog of cognac and whisky. The strangeness of the Dissecting Room, its unspeakable sights all marinated in the indelible stink of formalin. He had not been the only novitiate to rush from the room that first morning and throw up. There had been cold pork for dinner at home that night, weirdly—but also brought up, warmer, later.

"Such a sensitive boy," his mother had often defended him to his father.

"Made of sterner stuff now," he murmured, drunkenly, to his mute traveling companion.

And felt an immediate, slight catch in his throat. It seemed a sad thing, that lost sensitivity. Where had it vanished? Or had it, in fact, vanished? If he was sensitive enough to grieve for lost sensitivity, then surely he hadn't, in fact, lost it.

The paradox tickled him; he chuckled drunkenly, recovering already from the brief, foolish outbreak of sentimentality.

"Ladies and gentlemen, Captain Baker again from the flight deck. I realize the trip has been, ah, difficult for many of you, and I apologize for any inconvenience. As you will understand, the circumstances were beyond our control. But we have made good progress and will shortly be commencing our descent into Canberra."

Philip leaned forward and peered out through the Perspex window—nothing but cloud. The pressure on his bladder was becoming more urgent; in need of relief, he tried to rise from his aisle seat, but was jerked back. Something was gripping his waist; he strained against it, and was again tugged back. He glanced down. Of course. He released the seat belt clasp, and slid over into the middle seat.

"Excuse me," he said, and stood and lifted one leg over the dead man's leg, but failed to find solid ground on the far side, and unbalanced backward, finishing sprawled across the middle and window seats, an armrest pushing painfully into his back.

"Doctor?"

The purser was leaning in.

"Just in time," Philip said. "Another scotch, *danke schön.*"

"We've had some complaints, Doctor. Might I suggest something soft? And if you could fasten your seat belt."

"I'll fasten my seat belt," he said. "If you get me another scotch."

"I'm sorry, sir. That's not possible. But we'll be landing soon. And further refreshments will be available in the terminal."

"It's for my throat," Philip said. "A slight tickle. I need a scotch to soothe my throat."

He rearranged himself into a sitting position in the window seat; the purser calmly leaned across and fastened his seat belt. "Perhaps a nap, Doctor."

"If you read me a story, first," he said. "And I'd like one of those cute little coloring-in kits."

"Please, Doctor. I know it's difficult. But it won't be long."

Through rising giddiness, he remembered that he had meant to work during the flight. The first draft of his paper for the Trans-Tasman conference needed fine-tuning: "The Civic Duty to Die Cheaply." It was in his valise, wherever that was. His heavy eyelids slid shut, the giddiness worsened. Work was clearly beyond him, the title of his paper too absurd anyway, too comically unlikely.

He forced his eyes back open. Would Holly be waiting at the arrival gate? He hoped so; he suddenly felt in need of her physical presence. Her hands, her voice, her heart. Her warm heart. He reached for his mobile phone, still safely holstered on his belt, turned it on, and punched his home number. Was he in range? Apparently. The number was ringing.

"Hello?"

"Sweetheart? It's me. We're about to land. Where are you?"

A brief silence, then an icy voice, "Is that you, Philip? Are you drunk again?"

"Drunk with love."

The voice moved beyond iciness, into permafrost. "I won't be picking you up at the airport, Philip. This is Mary, not Holly. We've been divorced for five years, remember?"

The young attendant was again at his side. "Doctor, we don't permit the use of mobile phones while the aircraft is in flight. I must insist."

"Just a minute, Tight Lips. I'm in the middle of a conversation . . ."

But Mary had hung up. He chuckled at his absentmindedness. How had he managed to dial the old number? Ingrained habit? He remembered those first months after he had left Mary and the boys, of how he would often find himself parked outside the house, driving home from the hospital on autopilot, his mind elsewhere. He had never told Holly of these innocent episodes, sensing that she would be hurt, or would read some absurd deeper significance into them.

The purser's voice was suggesting preparations for landing. Philip obediently raised his seat, and the middle seat, but his companion's controls were beyond his reach.

"Please return your body to the upright position, sir," he said, and giggled.

The aircraft rocked, descending through cloud; one of Mr. Brice's hands flopped out from beneath the covering blanket, and onto the middle seat. Anything was suddenly possible. Philip, dazed, reached out and clasped it. The fingers were cold; he remembered again the room-temperature coldness of that first assigned corpse, years before. A woman of eighty, eighty-five. He remembered lifting the linen covering aside for the first time, terrified. He remembered the immense difficulty of making an initial incision into the white-leather skin. He had willed his trembling hand to move that day, to grasp the scalpel and cut. Then tease apart the tissues with his fingers—blunt dissection, in the argot. His thin gloves had done nothing to disguise the greasiness of the exposed flesh.

He squirmed, reliving his squeamishness. Who said he was insensitive—at least when he had been drinking? The smoky magic of scotch—it always found him out, sniffed out his dormant self like a dog. He had spent a year teasing that old lady apart, a year in which horror had slowly been replaced by fascination—and, finally, by awe. Was he getting sentimental again? About a corpse? Better sentimental than squeamish. Such a marvelous structure, that frail body. Form so perfectly matched to function. And—he smiled to himself, remembering—with a spare of everything packed in. Lungs, kidneys, ovaries. Hands, feet. Ears. Eyeballs.

A spare of everything, at any rate, except a heart.

The rumble of landing gear being lowered distracted him from his drunken reverie. The itch had left his throat, but there was surely time for one last drink. He reached up his hand and pressed the call button. No response. He pressed again, and when there was again no response, apart from that tiny red light, kept his finger pushed against the button, firmly.

Finding Joshua

JACINTA HALLORAN

It is not so much a question of leaving. The question "Why leave?" demands the justification of action: the packing of a suitcase, the severing of habit. But consider the question "Why stay?" Now everything is turned on its head. You must then find a reason for waking each morning next to someone you no longer know. You must justify the silences that stretch for days at a time, the sudden tightness in your chest as you hear his car in the driveway. In matters such as these, it's important to ask the right questions.

We live the life of ghosts now, David and I. In the evenings, after dinner—a can of soup, a frozen lasagna: the meals cooked by friends and left at the doorstep have long since petered out—I retire to the TV, David to his study. Late at night, I often hear the click of the study latch and his footsteps in the hall. He moves from room to room, his footfall hesitant, as if he is searching for something misplaced. I hear him enter Joshua's room and I turn up the TV volume so that my eardrums ache. Some nights he doesn't come to bed. I do not ask him where he sleeps, or if he sleeps at all. Perhaps, like the ghosts we now resemble, he wanders the house until morning, communing with bricks and mortar, waiting for the house to yield up its secrets. In Joshua's room, there must be secrets yet to be revealed: words scratched into the desk; a coded cipher in the arrangement of books on the shelf; somewhere, somehow a last-minute message of absolution. *It is not your fault.*

My psychiatrist tells me it is natural to feel guilty, that guilt is part of grieving. Of course I know this—I have read the literature, counseled my share of bereaved patients—but the knowledge I possess is of a cold, uncomforting kind. It does nothing to drown out those questions that clamor, demanding answers, at 3:00 a.m. The facts and statistics—what I used to call my training—stubbornly reside in my head, unable to soothe me to sleep, powerless to release the squeezing of my heart or slow my hungry breathing. I used to be arrogant enough to think I was prepared for grief.

I have gone back to work. Where else is there to go? I work for as long as I can, but usually by lunchtime my head throbs so badly I cannot continue. It is then that I put away my stethoscope and, with a nod to Margaret or Jill at Reception, I leave the clinic, impervious to the irritation of the patients who sit there, still waiting to see me. I'm surprised I am able to leave when there is work still to be done—such uncharacteristic behavior—but then, nothing is as it was. Besides, it's unwise to consult when the headaches are at their peak. The pain robs me of my train of thought and the nausea can bring me to my knees. As the morning progresses and the headache builds, my thoughts become loose, my short-term memory impaired, as if the pain itself were a toxic substance, seeping through the brain, leaving countless damaged neurons in its wake. I find myself gazing out the window or doodling as my patients talk. To help with concentration, I write down their complaints verbatim in their files, but when they have left the room, I stare at these dictated phrases, no longer able to extract their meaning. I suppose these are migraines, though I have also wondered if I have a brain tumor; have, at times, almost wished for a disease that carried with it the tantalizing promise of a permanent amnesia. At other times, I hate myself for such thoughts. If I forfeit memory, what else is there?

I hear all the time of children dying: burned in house fires, the parents absent; killed in car accidents; drowned in backyard pools; teenagers who climb on top of moving trains and slam into bridges at eighty kilometers an hour. *I am not alone,* I tell myself, as another story of loss is splashed across the newspaper or the television screen. *There are many mothers like me.* I have looked for comfort in such thoughts, but I have come to realize there is no comfort to be gleaned from the suffering of others. Now, in the evenings, instead of watching news or current affairs, I lie on the couch—I have it all to myself—soaking up sitcoms and soapies, quiz shows, and talent quests. I'm sustained by the banal and the bland, the soporific and the ridiculous: there is nothing like television to deaden the mind.

As a doctor, I have learned to watch and listen as my patients speak, taking note of not only their words, but also the unconscious messages they send. Subtle shifts in body language, the vagaries of affect and mood, the Freudian slip of the tongue: these are the secret tools of my trade. After twenty years of practice, such things were instinctive, or so I thought. But with Joshua, it seems my instinct deserted me. When did I stop taking note of my son? His infant milestones, his primary school years are clear in my mind; years of simple needs and simple pleasures. I can still see him, aged twelve, on the first day of secondary school: kicking at the front steps, trying to dull the shine on his new black shoes, the sleeves of his blazer hanging down to his knuckles. In the early hours of the morning, when I have given up all hope of sleep, I stand at the kitchen window and relive his thirteenth birthday party: a warm summer's evening, the *thwack* of the bouncing trampoline, the husky banter of adolescent boys, the verandah table laden with food and drink. ("Not healthy stuff, Mum," he had begged me. "We've got to have pizzas and loads of soft drinks.") In the muted light of early evening, David moved around the garden in his methodical way, taking photos of Josh with each of his friends. I insisted we sing "Happy Birthday." Was I hopelessly misguided? Now, at the kitchen window, my dressing gown drawn tight against the cold, I close my eyes, trying to recall the expression on Josh's face as he bent down to blow out the thirteen candles, but the edges of memory start to blur. I can no longer be sure what I remember or what, with hindsight, I've insinuated into the picture. Were there shadows even then? I fast-forward to this year, but his face shifts out of focus and turns away from my gaze. When was the last time I took his face in my hands and brushed the hair from his eyes? When did he become the ghost of himself, noiseless and ephemeral, slipping through my fingers?

Somewhere in this empty house, the photographs of that birthday lie neatly framed in one of David's albums. In other albums, on shelves and in cupboards, are other photos of other times, taking their rightful place alongside school reports, homemade birthday cards, basketball trophies, swimming medallions. Drawers that I dare not open, crammed with tokens of the past. Is this the measure of sixteen years?

I have not seen Josh's friends since the funeral. I understand their reluctance to visit us in our mausoleum, to sit in our neglected garden with the rusting trampoline. They are young: their place is with the living. Besides, they know there are questions to be answered, questions they would rather avoid. They are young but they may not be blameless. Some of them harbor secrets, kept safe too long. After the service, as they filed past me one by one—the boys red-eyed, with shoulders hunched; the girls weeping openly—I searched each face for answers. If I could have found voice I would have asked the boys, *Which of you knew and did not tell?* Someone must have known. And of the girls: *Which of you broke his heart?* But perhaps Josh was born with a broken heart: a hairline fracture, a congenital weakness that I did not detect and, consequently, failed to mend.

David's hands still shake. At the dinner table, between each mouthful of food, he presses his palms together, as if in prayer. I watch as he separates his hands and blows lightly on each open palm, as if he can still feel the burning coarseness of the rope against his fingers. I have given him sedatives but he does not take them. He is on his own. There is nothing I can do.

It was David who found him. It was David who untied the rope and felt the weight of Josh's body against his. It was David who knelt at his side when the paramedics ceased resuscitation. And it was David, not me, who first ran his hands down Josh's limp arms, tracing with his fingers the myriad lines, some healed as the faintest of scars, some cut only days before. I was still at work, attending to my patients. I didn't know. David hadn't phoned me. By the time I got home it was all over. My son's illness and death were over.

Does it matter now? Of course David was in shock. He didn't think. It was only fifteen minutes—twenty, at the most—before he called to let me know. Would it have made a difference if I had been there earlier? Having failed for sixteen years to save my son, could I have saved him then?

These questions hang in the air between us, echoing through every room in this house of horrors. In my silence, I ask them of David. In his silence, he reproaches me for asking. Never before has it mattered that I am a doctor and David is not. Does it matter now? It's the only thing that matters.

Why, then, do I stay? Because I have come to believe in the possibility of ghosts. Because I must stay until I no longer believe.

Memories are ghosts of a kind: specters that haunt without sound or vision, terrorizing our sleep, tormenting our waking hours. In my work, I have seen what damage memories can do. I have one memory—of course there are many—but one that haunts me most of all. I recount it to my psychiatrist at each weekly visit. She, in her dispassionate way, tells me I am imbuing the story with added meaning; that, in short, I am overreacting. I do not believe her.

It was early autumn: the faintest of chills in the afternoon air, the leaves of the plane trees just beginning to turn. I'd picked Josh up from kindergarten and as we walked home I asked him, as all mothers do in their less inspired moments, "So, what did you do today?"

He kicked at a stone on the path and did not reply. I persisted. "Who did you play with? What did you make? Did the teacher read a story?"

He looked at me, then, with those wide blue eyes that could appear almost vacant: a trick of his, a way he had, from an early age, of deflecting the outside world. "You are asking all the wrong questions," he said. He was three years old.

I used to tell this as a humorous anecdote, an example of my son's precociousness, a gentle ribbing of myself as the distracted, inattentive mother. Because, at the time, I didn't really believe I was inattentive. But now the story seems glaring in its omissions. Now it is a story of negligence. Surely you see what is missing. The question I now ask myself every hour of every day, because I never thought to ask it of him: "Tell me, Josh, what are the right questions?"

What, my darling boy, were the right questions?

Tahirih

LEAH KAMINSKY

I stand at the entrance to the waiting room. Tahirih looks up and smiles, waiting patiently for me, hands folded in her lap.

"Come in, Tahirih," I say.

Tahirih smoothes the creases from her tailored navy skirt. Her eyebrows sculpted, her graying hair scraped back into a neat bun, she wears a silk blouse and her pumps are white. Silhouetted against the sunlight bleeding in through the wooden shutters of the waiting room, she looks like she is wearing a halo.

"I don't mind waiting," she says. "You can take that man in before me. He is so distressed."

"Thank you, Tahirih, but let's get started, shall we?"

The morning they called Tahirih to the morgue in Tehran, she asked the caretaker if she could wash Fouad's body. She told me that her husband had always been such a clean and elegant man and she could not stand to see him lying on a steel table, covered in blood and excrement. The caretaker brought her a bucket of water and an old rag. This was the body that belonged to her all those years, the body of which she had once been so shy.

Tahirih was seventeen when she first met Fouad. Her

mother called her away from piano practice to introduce her to some visitors. She was annoyed at the interruption. When she walked into the living room, she saw him seated beside his mother. They were all sipping cherry juice, a delicacy served only on special occasions. It was a hot day and Tahirih was feeling a little faint as she stood before everyone.

"Come sit with us," her mother said. "I want you to meet Mrs. Faizi and her son Fouad. They are here visiting from Tehran for a short while." Tahirih sat down on the edge of an armchair.

"Would you care for some fresh dates or figs?" her mother asked, passing a tray of delicacies across to Mrs. Faizi. Fouad stared at Tahirih. She looked away. Two red roses stood in a vase on the coffee table. Her mother had cut some of her prize flowers from the garden. That signaled that these visitors were very important. Tahirih had certainly heard of Mrs. Faizi before. Her husband was a member of the Baha'i Spiritual Assembly in Tehran, but Tahirih had never known that they had a son.

"Fouad is an engineer," her mother said. "He is visiting his parents for a few days, and they have kindly come up to see us today." Tahirih nodded, thinking only about her piano exam the following week. Her mother handed her a plate of almonds to offer the guests. She smiled politely and placed it on the table in front of Fouad. Their eyes met briefly again, and this time he smiled. He had a dark mustache, streaked with gray, which made him look quite handsome.

"I heard you playing before," he said. " 'Für Elise' is one of my favorite pieces."

Tahirih picked up her glass and brought it to her lips before realizing that it was empty.

"Would you play some more for me?" he asked.

"Oh, um . . ." were the only words she could push past her tongue before her mother interrupted.

"Of course she will." Tahirih could see that her mother was eager to please this man. "It would be an honor, wouldn't it, Tahirih?" She urged her daughter to get up, holding her hand out in the direction of the parlor.

Tahirih stood up and turned to go. At the same time, Fouad rose from the sofa.

She felt him following her as she walked slowly into the other room. He closed the curtain behind them and stood leaning against the wall. The music rose up, breaking the awkward silence. Minute after minute passed as her fingers pawed at the keys, the tune a muted drone in the background compared to her pounding heart. As she finished playing the last bars, the notes sank away into silence and Fouad sighed. He walked over to where Tahirih was seated and stood behind her, placing his hands on her shoulders. She felt his warm breath on the back of her neck.

"You are lovely," he whispered.

Tahirih remembers the day her daughter Bahiya was born, how her tiny fingers curled around her mother's thumb, her head tossing as she rooted around for the nipple. She once told me that they sent her a bill for the bullets the firing squad used to execute her husband. They came in the middle of the night and dragged him out of bed. The last time she saw him, a sliver of moonlight shone between the slats of the shutters onto his back. She remembers thinking that she should have mended the hole in his pajama shirt. Her mind still clutches at that loose thread, as if it still ties their destiny together. It is as long as it needs to be, winding through her years like an intricate, silken web across the globe. She never thought then that it would lead her to Haifa.

She hid the account for the bullets in the hem of her dress when she was smuggled out of Tehran after Fouad was killed. She still keeps it in a special box in the top drawer of her bedside table, opening it from time to time, usually just before she goes to bed. She runs her fingers over the faded print. She has to touch it, to prove that it is real. Ten bullets fired into his chest. The bill was dated 4/21/1979 and sent by the Iranian Ministry of Finance, account payable in thirty days. She also received monthly bills for "food and accommodation."

Here in Haifa, she tells me that people are kind to her. The Arab girl at the kiosk blesses her in Hebrew every day. The tiny Jewish lady in the apartment opposite greets her every morning as she beats a rug over the balcony rail.

"*Ah'lan!*" her neighbor shouts. "Everything will be fine, God willing." *Tfoo, tfoo, tfoo,* the woman spits to ward off the evil eye.

She has a job in archives at the Baha'i World Centre. Baha'is visit from all over the world to work as volunteers, and each one has a tale to tell. They treat her well and look after her every need. She repays their kindness by working hard. She believes that work is worship.

The lady in a fur coat steps slowly off the bus every morning, carrying a mop in her hand. Winter or summer, she smiles at her and walks on. This land of contradictions is Tahirih's home now. Her friend Katya has thrown away her wedding ring. She told her she stood completely naked in front of the mirror one morning and felt that part of her had been born while another part had died. After throwing away the golden band that had been part of her body for twenty-five years, she felt free.

And as Tahirih tells me this, I clutch onto my own wedding band, while Tahirih fiddles with the invisible thread tied to her ring, forever joined to Fouad. But somehow, the more she tugs, the further the thread unravels. Tahirih remains married to a dead man.

Tahirih said they came in the night, knocked loudly, then kicked the door in just as she was about to get up. She was home alone with Bahiya. Fouad had already been in prison a month by then. The tall one was chewing sunflower seeds. He smiled at her and ran his fingers through his black, greasy hair. One of his front teeth was missing, and through the gap he spat the cracked shells onto the Persian rug in the living room. He motioned with his right hand to the guard who accompanied him. The young soldier left the room and went outside.

The ugly one stayed. He walked his huge hand over the spines of the books on the bookshelf, like a concert pianist practicing his scales.

"It seems that you are very clever," he laughed, pulling Bahiya's favorite book down from the shelf: *Little Red Riding Hood*. "Is this one of your filthy infidel books?" he asked as he stroked the picture of the little girl on the cover.

The ugly one was still smiling as he slowly tore each page. He ripped Little Red Riding Hood to pieces and threw her severed head onto the floor. He ran his fingers along the spines of the books on the shelf again, and pulled one out, asking her to read him the title.

"Don't dare lie, you prostitute," he said quietly, "or I will kill you here and now."

"God is my witness that I will not lie to you."

"Shut up!" He shoved her to the ground. "Don't mention the name of God with your filthy mouth."

He lowered his black army boot onto her hair. He kneeled down and smiled at her, like someone had flicked a switch in his brain. He turned away, his attention wandering back to the bookshelves. He lifted the butt of his rifle this time and pointed to the Koran.

"Why is this your shelf?"

"It is a Holy book," she began, "the Baha'is honor its wisdom and—"

"Bow down to Allah and save your soul."

She stared down at the rug. He continued looking through the books. That particular evening, the third time they had visited unannounced since her husband's arrest, it was to be one of Fouad's textbooks. The guard pointed to a paragraph and sat down on the couch, patting the cushions and motioning for Tahirih to sit next to him.

She started to read out loud, just as if little Bahiya was seated by her side and they were reading a bedtime story. *The phenomenon called migratory crystallization consists in the growth of large crystals in a group, at the expense of small ones. The response of the system to invasion by ice molecules determines the immediate and long-term effects of freezing.*

"It is such a warm and pleasant night," he said.

Her heart was pounding. He slowly tore out the page she had been reading and scrunched it up into a ball. He handed it to her and said: "Eat it."

She did not move.

"Go on. Eat some ice to cool you down."

She took the paper from his outstretched hand. She was trembling so much that she accidentally dropped it on the floor.

"Pick it up."

She bent down, and he suddenly grabbed her wrist and forced her down onto her knees. His right hand held the back of her head firmly by the roots of her hair. He rose above her, unzipped the trousers of his dirty uniform and forced himself into her mouth, thrusting as she gagged and choked. When he finished, he threw her back onto the floor and she landed on top of a photo of Baha'u'llah. She vomited bile and semen onto his Holy face.

She looked up for a moment toward Bahiya's room and thought she saw a tiny shadow disappear back into the darkness of the hallway. The books on the shelf started to whirl around her head; the guard's laughter echoed in her ears.

I ask Tahirih to lift her blouse and place my cold stethoscope on her skin. "Breathe in," I say automatically.

Usually the air rushing in and out of healthy lungs sounds like waves washing up onto shore then receding. Sometimes I lose focus when I examine a patient's chest, and don't seem to register what I am actually hearing. Today, the gurgling rattle of Tahirih's lungs won't let my mind wander very far. I put down my stethoscope and scribble out a form for a chest X-ray.

"Always better to play it safe," I say matter-of-factly, as she tucks in her blouse. I hand her the referral.

"Bless you, doctor, for squeezing me in," Tahirih says, reaching out and touching my hand lightly. "I would be grateful if you would give me something for this cough, meanwhile, just to help me sleep a little at night."

I pull my hand away from hers just a little too quickly, and try to cover up my embarrassment by scribbling out a prescription for some antibiotics. The infernal itch is back. Every month I douse the bastards and every month they set up shop in my hair. Oh, the joys of motherhood.

"Thank you, doctor," Tahirih says. She is so accepting.

Most patients nowadays ask me endless questions, pull out some crap they've printed off the Internet, wanting to discuss the results of the latest trials of the inhibition of IM-9 leukocyte 3-hydroxy-3-methylglutaryl coenzyme, which I've never even heard of. They think their cybersurfing gives them an instant medical degree. I just don't get it. Why are they so willing to swallow hocus-pocus herbs from some witch doctor without giving it a second thought, yet demand that I explain all the side effects and possible risks of anything and everything I prescribe? A simple *thank you, doctor* once in a while comes as such a relief. They have lost their faith in the profession, so that life in this room usually boils down to plumbing and pills. I am tired of listening. I am bloated with their stories. I have nowhere left to put them anymore. They spill out from me onto the pavement as I walk down the street, and I seem to be losing pieces of myself along the way.

I am beginning to forget myself lately as well. Maybe it's the pregnancy? More often than not, while a patient is in the midst of unfolding his or her life to me, I doodle on prescription pads, or prepare shopping lists, my mind edging slowly toward the door and out. I am always waiting for the opportunity to go to the bathroom while a patient undresses. I leave the room and escape from those voices that constantly beg *help me, mend me*. I stand there, staring into the mirror at a face I barely recognize anymore. And as I turn away from the sink, telling myself to get a grip and go back in to the patient waiting for me, I catch a glimpse of someone else walking off in the opposite direction, into the depths of the mirror. This doppelganger of mine is never coming back. The Mirror Woman peels off her white coat like dead skin and heads down to the sea. I go back into my room and start searching for pathology.

Listen to me carrying on! I am supposed to dispense compassion and humanity along with the pills, to be a healer, a listener, a therapist, a fixer, a priest, a mother, a confidante, a bloody miracle worker for all of them. The truth is, I'm tired. I have been there for all the important milestones. I have stood beside freshly dug graves as they are buried, listening to the words of the Kaddish over and over again. I have walked alone in cemeteries and wept for those I could not save, or for those I could have saved, should have saved but didn't. But the truth is, I am secretly weeping for myself, for my own mortality.

I move over to the washbasin by the window. I rinse my hands with chlorhexidene disinfectant; a well-programmed robot, I wash slowly, thoroughly, rubbing my palms together in a circular motion, cleaning meticulously between the fingers with the scrubbing brush. A tiny black louse is lodged under the nail of my right index finger. I quickly flick it out, and it drops into the basin. I watch it swirl around in the opposite direction to what it would in Melbourne, and finally it disappears down the drain.

How can I know how to help Tahirih? She is filled with forgiveness and love and understanding for everyone, even for the very people who hated and abused her.

"I did not want to trouble you again today, dearest doctor," she says. "You are so busy with people who need your help far more than me. I am so sorry to bother you."

She notices me shifting around on my chair.

"You are not comfortable?"

"I'm fine, Tahirih." I hold a hand to my lower back and fend off her intrusion. "It's just the pregnancy. I haven't been sleeping so well lately."

"Doctor," she says, "I hope you don't mind me saying this, but you have been looking quite tired lately. I am a little worried."

"I wish I was more like you," I say. "Where can I buy such patience and acceptance?"

She clutches at her necklace of freshwater pearls, and I watch her mouth as it moves.

"Baha'u'llah says the actions of those that persecute us are born out of innocence."

Something about her reminds me of an old wooden ventriloquist's doll I used to have as a child.

"It's always best," she says, trying to stifle a cough, "to kiss your killer's hand."

I hope she won't notice as I reach up to scratch my scalp.

Communion

JOHN MURRAY

Her father was put in her bed, the big mahogany bed that had come over from Germany. Elsbeth went to sleep on a portable bed in Charlie's room. In the end, her father would not sleep with her mother. He refused to sleep with her. By then his nature, his whole being, had changed. He flailed his arms, shouted, laughed for no reason, sometimes sang songs. When Elsbeth went into the room, he watched her silently from the bed like a caged animal. She tried reading to him, sections from the Bible or *Tom Sawyer* that he liked, but he shouted for her to stop after a few pages. This was in the ninth week. For the first eight weeks, he was still himself, able to walk around, but nauseated and dizzy when he stood up. Still, he pulled on his clothes in the morning and went out with her grandfather. They were bringing in the corn then, and her father tried to do the work he had always done. He was exhausted by lunchtime and had to come in and lie down on the sofa, sleeping for the rest of the afternoon with his head back and his palms outstretched—strange and otherworldly with the front of his head shaved, like a mental patient. The neurosurgeon had shaved the hair off the front of his head, up to the crown, so he could open up his skull. A piece of his brain had been taken out and looked at under a microscope. This was in the teaching hos-

pital in Minneapolis, the university hospital, where he had
been taken from the church.

Her father had collapsed during Sunday Mass. Charlie
had begun screaming, and her father had to take him back
through the church. She heard him talking to Charlie outside, carrying him up and down the path alongside the
church, his shoes crunching loudly on the gravel. That was
why he was the last to receive the Communion—everyone
else had already sat down when he came in along the aisle,
handed Charlie to her mother, and went forward to Father
Figge. He was halfway up the aisle when he collapsed. He
made a sighing sound, a long, loud yawn, and then fell to
his knees. It almost seemed like an act of worship, like
something connected with the ceremony. But the sound was
wrong—it became a moan, a gasping sound, too loud and
too long, and then her father fell sideways. His head struck
the stone floor with a sound like a bowling ball dropped on
cement—an unnatural sound. And for a moment the con-
gregation, that church full of people, did nothing but watch,
amazed, in awe perhaps. Father Figge stood holding the cup
and the bread, his mouth hanging open, and the church was
filled with a rhythmic sound of her father on the cold stone
floor, eyes rolled up, jaw clenched, back arched, arms and
legs stiff and thrashing, a dark stain appearing on the front
of his pants like a curse, an irregular spreading stain shaped
like a map—North America, South America, Continental
Europe, and beyond.

It was Floss Melcher who knew what to do. She said loudly
that he was having a fit, and ran out to get a stick to put
between his teeth. His jaw was clenching and unclenching,

and there was blood around his lips. She brought a piece of cherry-blossom wood, got down on her knees, and forced it between his lips with difficulty. He was working and thrashing on the ground, grunting like an animal, his face dusky. Floss also asked two of the men to roll him carefully onto his side, so that he would be able to breathe. Charlie began screaming. Her mother kneeled next to her father with one hand on his shoulder, trying to keep him down, still wearing her white hat with the false lilies around the edge, holding her handbag in the elbow of one arm. Father Jewett appeared to be praying, muttering words under his breath. Five minutes later, her father stopped jerking and lay still, breathing lightly through blue lips, unconscious. Four men took hold of his arms and legs and carried him out to the car park. Ern Wiltstein had backed up his Chrysler. They put him flat along the backseat, knees bent, arm hanging down lifeless on the floor. Decisions were made quickly. At that time there was no ambulance service in town and no hospital either, so they knew they had to drive to the city. Her mother rode with Ern Wiltstein. Someone decided that Charlie should go home with her grandfather. Floss took Elsbeth and said they would ride down to the hospital together; stopped on the way for ice cream, a cherry soda, peppermint chewing gum, and a pack of cigarettes.

Elsbeth did not want to turn away. She saw this about herself. She wanted to know, to see everything under bright fluorescent lights. She needed to have details, facts, the hard and practical truth. This was in her and always would be. She went with Floss to the white hospital room where her father had woken up, as if from a deep sleep. He was groggy and disoriented. He looked around the room as if he had never seen a room before. But to see him awake filled Elsbeth with confidence. She imagined that she had caused him to wake up by will alone. She stood in the corner of the hospital room and felt a kind of satisfaction. The nurses, clean and rasping in their starched uniforms and tight white stockings, moved around the room. They managed to get her father into a hospital smock (he could not lift his arms or legs properly), then took blood from his arm with a needle and large glass syringe, measured his pulse, temperature, and blood pressure. All of these measurements, the fact of them, seemed to make her father's condition manageable. Elsbeth wanted to reassure her mother. But her mother was unreachable—terrified. She stood away from the bed, did not touch Elsbeth's father, barely spoke. She looked young, like a girl dressed up in adult clothes—awkward and ordinary. When they took her father out of the room for a series of tests (X-rays of the skull, an angiogram, an electroencephalogram—Elsbeth was later to learn all of these terms), her mother sat down on the edge of a seat with her handbag in her lap and shook. Floss kneeled next to her on the floor and said she had a cousin who had fits, she had seen it before. She knew it could be controlled with tablets. It was possible for people to get on with their lives.

"You don't just get fits," her mother said.

"I don't know."

"You don't just get them."

The room was a public room containing three other beds, but only one of the beds was occupied. An old man lay on this bed reading a newspaper. He held the paper up in front of his face and turned the pages loudly. Below, both lower legs lay out on top of the bed, fat and white, and there were bandages around his feet. Elsbeth could see that the feet were too short—the toes had been removed, so that his feet had become stubs. When he turned the pages of the paper, the old man looked at Elsbeth and she saw that one of his eyes did not open—he stared at her with his good eye, a malicious and angry stare, and she stared back. She could not be daunted, felt willing to see terrible things. She would not allow anything to shock her.

From the window, the hospital room overlooked a construction site. A crane was lifting long steel girders up onto a steel platform that had already been built. Men in white hats and leather gloves stood at the top, steadying the long pieces of steel as they swayed slowly onto the platform; through the thick glass Elsbeth could hear the distant rumble of the machines, the clang of the materials. Over the next three days, she would see the building take shape, the girders bolted into each other to form a frame, walls put into place, steady progress. The building rose from the ground, just as her father faded from it, slipped slowly from view, became a series of technical terms that carried nothing but an abstract weight.

Glioblastoma. This was what they called it. A tumor, a mass. Inoperable. It was taking over his brain, the frontal and parietal lobes, exploding silently and invisibly beneath his skull. It had caused him to lose his sense of smell. It had caused the seizure. It would continue to grow. It would cause building pressure inside the cranial vault. This was the term the neurosurgeon had used—cranial vault. The neurosurgeon was a short man with a scrubbed pink face who talked slowly. A day later, he did surgery under a general anesthetic. He took out as much of the tumor as he reasonably could—decompressed it, he said—then patched it all up again and put back the bone. He came to see her mother while her father was still unconscious. He led her away along the corridor to a small glass office with carpet the color of gravy. He had beautiful hands. Pink sculpted fingers and clean fingernails. He pointed at a large wall-poster of the brain and skull in cross section, and another showing the effects of a tumor. That was when he used the term cranial vault. An expanding mass inside the cranial vault, he said. A glioblastoma. Aggressive. Quite beyond medical science. Months seemed possible, weeks more likely. It was all about pressure. They would work to keep the pressure down, but eventually this would not be possible and the brain would be squeezed out of the cranial vault entirely. There was no easy way to put it, he had never believed in creating false hope. Did he notice that Elsbeth had followed them down the corridor and stood behind her mother? It did not seem likely. She wore her pink lacy dress, pink headband, white kneesocks (still held up with elastics), smelled of coffee, perfume. It was she who caught her mother when she fell, put her arms behind her back, and lowered her to the floor with difficulty, looked down at her makeup-smudged face and told the neurosurgeon to go away. She kneeled over her mother, pulled the hair away from her face, took off the white hat with false lilies carefully and put it on the floor, found her handkerchief (white, starched, folded in quarters), and wiped her mother's eyes, cheeks, and mouth with the precision of an undertaker. She put her mother's head in her lap and kept her eyes on the technical diagrams on the wall, repeated the terms she saw there as if they would somehow make a difference.

A nurse came in to look after her father. This was always done in the country—the nurse came and lived in the house and took care of the sick person. The nurse was Elsbeth's aunt on her father's side—her father's sister, only three years older. Her name was Lily, and she had married a farmer named Ralph Bittner. They lived on a farm a hundred miles to the south and were poor. All her father's siblings—two girls (Lily and Esther) and a boy (Henry)—were poor. Elsbeth grew up slightly frightened of them. They were lean, hard people who did not smile. They visited at Thanksgiving and Christmas, brought gifts of food—a haunch of ham, a basket of fresh carrots and potatoes, three woodcock tied together by the feet. It was not possible to please or flatter them with words or gestures. They made Elsbeth feel as if she knew too much. She felt certain that they resented her mother for being happy and talkative, for her books and modern dresses, and for her choice to abandon a comfortable life in town for farm life, a life they struggled through. Lily had caught the state bus all the way north, then a local bus out along the main road. She walked from the main road with her suitcase.

Lily took charge, swept everything before her. She was a doer. She had trained as a nurse, then given it up to go on the farm with Ralph and have two children, raise them, do the work of a man during the harvest, develop a problem in her womb that made her so anemic that she needed a transfusion and then a hysterectomy. Now she propped them up with piecework as a home nurse, of which there was "plenty, make no mistake, plenty as need it, make no mistake." She was paid to do this work, although payment was never discussed. The payment took place at the end—an envelope, usually, passed over shyly, imperceptibly, as she moved out the door.

She slept in the dining room on the ground floor. This had always been the fancy room of the house. It had a polished mahogany table, an oak sideboard with a mirror, a marble mantelpiece with an anniversary clock, and a pot filled with peacock feathers. A carved bust of Venus and a small abstract shape by Henry Moore sat on the sideboard.

The curtains were red velvet and tied with a sash. On winter days, her mother sat at the table and polished her silver cutlery, arranging the pieces next to each other in long rows, taking a kind of pride in the different types of spoons: tea, dessert, serving, soup, coffee, sugar. A bed was carried in and the table was moved to one side. Lily unpacked her suitcase and arranged her things along the tabletop: two textbooks (one of anatomy, another of general medicine); a stethoscope and a blood-pressure machine; an otoscope and an ophthalmoscope; a thermometer in a thin metal case; a watch with a chain that could be pinned to clothes; a Bible; two back issues of *Reader's Digest;* five bobby pins; two plastic tortoiseshell hair combs; a jar of Pond's skin cream; one toothbrush and one tube of toothpaste; one white nursing uniform and a pair of white shoes; one set of civilian clothes—a baggy floral day dress with a cloth belt and a pair of flat black shoes; one beige hat; three pairs of underwear; one slip; one bra; one nightgown (pink rayon); and one robe (also pink rayon) with shiny cuffs and collar. She hung the clothes on coat hangers from the mantel. Elsbeth studied these belongings carefully when her aunt was out. There was almost nothing personal about them, nothing to indicate that her aunt was an ordinary person. And she did not see herself as an ordinary person, this became clear. She thought of herself as superior.

"It's a crime you got out there," Lily said to her mother. "Still have the outdoor facility. Women like us should demand something modern. Those facilities is a hazard and not good for the health, and you can't expect us modern women, as knows something better, to keep on using them."

Us. Modern women. That was how she saw herself. Elsbeth was sure that Lily had brought the textbooks just for show; she never opened the books. Her superiority came from her power as a nurse, her secret knowledge. She saw it as her role to take over. She gave her mother a long list of items she would need from the stores in town (new pillows and sheets, a plastic bedcover, powders and rubs, meat). She put her father in Elsbeth's room and arranged bowls of water and cloths, syringes and needles, cotton wool and rubbing alcohol and medicines, then took over the washing and cooking. She believed in three square old-fashioned meals a day. Old-fashioned meals involved frying or roasting—and did not involve vegetables or fruit. She spooned lard into the pan freely, fried bacon, eggs, slices of hard German sausage or black pudding for breakfast; a piece of fried bread or leftover roast from the night before for lunch; a roast with potatoes and perhaps corn or beans for dinner, and always a pudding. She kept a weather eye on Elsbeth and Charlie at the table, refused to let them get up and leave until they had cleaned their plates. Everything tasted like oil. The house began to smell of it. This is what Elsbeth associated with Lily—the smell of oil on everything, and the slick, heavy food. It was food her grandfather liked, and he told his daughter so.

"Good to have real food," he said to Lily. "Real food is better for you."

"That's well known, Father," Lily said.

Everything was done in the white uniform. Elsbeth heard Lily get up before it was light, heard her washing in the kitchen, then walking to the outhouse. Some days, Lily chopped cordwood by the barn early, *thunk, thunk,* a shifting white shape at dawn—coming back quickly across the yard in her white shoes with a load for the stove. She washed the uniform and her underwear every night, at the laundry tub, rubbing hard with washing soap and a wire-bristled brush, rinsing and wringing, then hanging the clothes in front of the kitchen stove to dry overnight. And on Mondays she did all the washing, without being asked, starting before dawn, head down, arms working, not looking up or talking until it was all done and strung on the lines outside. She took control of the house. This left her mother in the position of having to accommodate Lily. Her mother baked and made tea and worked in the garden and felt awkward. She had never actually "run" a house in the same way, never had schedules or ways of doing things, nor had she cared to. She sat at the kitchen table with Lily and tried to engage her in conversation. Lily drank hot tea quickly, with her pinkie held out; wore her watch pinned to her breast and checked it constantly; kept the stethoscope, when she was inside, dangling around her neck as another trophy of her status. They talked about anything, everything, except what was really happening to her father. Death was a subject never discussed, although it was as vivid and present in that house as the floor and ceiling. This was the key to Lily—a hard-nosed avoidance of the truth in the guise of work. In front of her mother, Lily became a lady, talked about the garden, her children, played a kind of genteel game. When she got Elsbeth alone, she let down her guard and was quickly critical.

"A girl of your age should do more, I say that. Clothes washing you should do, and you can change the beds, look after the baby as well, take the load off of your mother. Your age, I was doing barn work, with no complaint, as well as caring for young children, because I had no mother. You understand? My mother went and died. I seen you. Don't think I haven't. I seen you lying around doing nothing."

They were outside pegging laundry on the line. Lily kept

working and did not look at Elsbeth, and said, "You got the curse yet? I got mine when I was twelve years old, painful as all get out, every month of my life. I know why they call it the curse—and I'll tell you what—the day I got my hysterectomy was the best day of my life. It's like a burden removed, make no mistake."

"Not yet."

"Well, you will."

It was in Elsbeth's nature to find fault, to undermine. She hated Lily quietly, did not believe her. There was no superiority there, she knew that, only bitterness. She saw it in Lily's threadbare clothes and in her red, shiny hands—red from the work. She saw it in her short, sharp movements when she plumped a pillow or made up a bed, or drew up the drugs (corticosteroids, diuretics, later pain medicine) from the little bottles with typed labels. Elsbeth watched her cleverly, listened to her sentences with scorn. Lily spoke in a way that country people spoke. It infuriated Elsbeth that her mother bowed down to Lily, tried to entertain and please her with cakes and conversations, praised her tirelessness and efficiency. Worse, her mother agreed to let Lily take over her father. She let Lily usher them out when she gave him injections; listened to her talking about him as if she knew better (no loud talk in his room, no singing, no discussion of anything that might be upsetting—the brain of the patient with a tumor is not a normal brain, Lily said, it's a brain that's all beaten up, and can't stand to be exerted). Even her father tried to flatter Lily, when he was still able. He teased her in the mornings, while Lily bustled about, cleaning and straightening. He spoke to her in the country way—not the way he spoke to her mother.

"I remember when Lily was a girl, maybe nineteen or twenty," he said. "Well, at that time there was young men from all over that wanted to go with her. You remember that, Lily?"

"I'm sure I do not remember."

"I remember very well, Lily. I remember one day in summer when there was two young men waiting in the yard in the morning to see you. You must remember that. Tony Nersesian and Gerald Volkmann—they were mad to see you. At that time you must have been out with both of them one or two times, to a dance or something. And then there they was one morning."

"That was a long time ago."

"Good-looking boys, they was, too. Good-looking and mad as bulls. Come down, Lily, they said, come down; we want you to choose between us, make one of us happy."

"Nothing special about either of them, neither."

"Well they was pretty strong for you, is all I can say. So you lean out of the window up here, like a princess, and look down on them and say, you'll go with the strongest, they'll have to fight it out. You don't care for boys who can't fight. You said that, and maybe you was kidding. But they took you on your word. All right, they said, so be it. Right down there in the yard, they pulled off their jackets and rolled up their sleeves, spit on their hands—and then they're away. It's nine o'clock in the morning, mind, and these two hammering away at each other, throwing punches. And Lily, calm as you like, is sitting up at the window laughing."

"You're exaggerating, Anton."

"Not exaggerating anything. Then they both got a few good punches in and there's some blood—and before you know it, one of them, I think it was Gerald Volkmann, was out cold on the ground, knocked out. The other one's not looking too good either, but he stood down there rubbing his hands and called up that he's yours. And cool as you like, you sat at the window and said that you've changed your mind, you prefer sensitive boys, not bloody fighters, because you're a pacifist."

"I never said pacifist."

Lily did not smile, but Elsbeth could see that she enjoyed being talked about. She kept going at the task at hand, but weakening and slowing down, wanting to prolong the moment. She did not seem to be her father's sister. They were more like acquaintances, talking freely with each other but showing no affection. This was another country way. And they looked different. Her father had big features, while Lily was fine boned with a small nose and mouth, made severe by her hair, which she pulled back in a bun. She wore no makeup and did not need any—her skin looked the same outside in bright light as it did inside.

Elsbeth blamed Lily for what was not acknowledged. They went on as if everything were normal. The steroids made her father put on weight. He walked outside. It was early winter now, and the ground was frozen hard in the mornings, the earth black, sometimes dusted with fine drifts of powdery snow. He wore a woollen cap over his shaved head. The scar from the operation had become a fine red line, and the skin over this area dipped down like a crater. He walked slowly and repeated the names of things he saw as if they were new to him: "That's the old barn," "There's the threshing machine," "There's the shed where we'd dress the hog carcasses." Elsbeth followed him around the yard hanging on to his sleeve, kept close to him, but said nothing. Her mother spent hours talking to him in the morning, and was always cheerful, laughing—her normal self. There was no indication that anything lay in wait. No preparations made. No fear. Elsbeth sat at the dining room table in the afternoon, white cloud and black frozen ground visible through the windows, and read the anatomy textbook, as if there were solutions to be found in diagrams of the cerebral hemispheres, or the cerebellum (leafy bulbs the texture of ornamental shrubs), or the convoluted arterial channels. But knowledge was a burden and did not help. The pictures of the flesh-colored interior landscape were as foreign and threatening as a primeval forest, the shores of an uncharted new land where the natives practiced cannibalism.

Very early one morning, Elsbeth heard her father going downstairs and outside before dawn. She dressed and went out after him. The car started in the shed. She kept out of sight behind the shed wall, and watched her father come out again and walk slowly back to the house. She went into the shed and got into the car, hunched down behind the driver's seat on the cold floor, and waited. Finally, her father came back, panting, got into the driver's seat heavily, and pulled out into the yard. He turned the heater up high and took off down the white road. It was still dark, a halo of light visible on the horizon. She kept low and watched the sky, power lines running past, listened to her father tapping the steering wheel, coughing. A few minutes later, the car bumped over some rough road and came to a stop. Through the window above her, she saw the black shapes of trees. Her father opened his window and she heard the rushing of water, and smelled the sour mud of the river. She waited for her father to get out, but he did not get out. He sat still in the front seat, not moving for five minutes, ten minutes. She heard him breathing. She crouched on the floor, her knees and ankles aching. Was he asleep? It seemed possible. She had decided to sit up and look around the seat, when he suddenly put the car into gear again and reversed back to the road. Twenty minutes later she felt the car run onto the sealed road, and in half an hour they were in town. A line of orange streetlights passed overhead, and then the car turned and came to a stop. Her father cracked open the door and got out. Elsbeth got out after him, coming to her feet suddenly. They were in the car park of Bruller's Diner, headlights passing on the road, the morning cold and still around them, the lights of the diner shining brightly. Her father did not see her at first. He was breathing heavily after getting out of the car, standing with his arms by his sides, looking around. She tugged on his sleeve. He bent down.

"Is that you, Tiger?"

"I came in the car."

"Well, I can see that, clear as day."

"I woke up early."

"Are you keeping an eye on me, Tiger?"

"I guess I am."

He took her hand and led her toward the diner. "I'm down here for breakfast, that's all. Come down for breakfast like I used to come. Just wanted to do it again."

They went inside. It was warm and smelled of coffee. The counter had a chrome edge and stools with red seats on silver poles. Two or three men sat eating at the counter. Ted Bruller was serving, wearing a long apron and a white cloth hat.

"Here's a surprise," he said.

"Missing your pancakes, Ted. Guess I brought the young'un down, too."

"You want pancakes and coffee. What about the little miss?"

"She can decide for herself."

"You allowed coffee?" Ted Bruller said to her.

"Let her have whatever she wants, Ted. My treat today."

The pancakes were irresistible—dark brown and spongy with a large rectangle of butter in the center, two rashers of bacon along the side, and fried potatoes. She put a spoonful of strawberry jam on top, and then the thick, warm maple syrup. And she had coffee, too, milky with sugar. She couldn't help but bolt it down, big mouthfuls of pancake and bacon and potato mixed together, and then mouthfuls of coffee as well. She wished she could have slowed down. Her father sat and took small bites with the tip of his fork; could not make headway. She watched him as he talked to Ted Bruller. In the harsh light of the diner, he looked sick; his skin white, his face and hands puffy. He did not take off his woolen cap—kept his scar covered. They talked about the price of corn and seed, the new machines that were coming in that year, the people he had known in school. Elsbeth felt as if this were a conversation she had heard many times before. The conversations would continue like this in the future, too, as monotonous and unending as the terrain. This was how people talked—in patterns. She cleaned her plate. Her father ate very little. He finally put down his fork and sat with his chin in his hands. He had drunk just half a cup of black coffee. Ted Bruller said there was no need to pay, it was on the house, but her father refused. He had never taken a free meal, he said, never would. He left the money on the counter.

"You thank Mr. Bruller, Tiger, for breakfast."

"No need to thank me, little miss. We'll see you again."

"See you again," her father said, and slid off the stool. "Keep well."

"You keep yourself well, Anton. Regards to Helen."

They went outside. The day had opened up, a beautiful fall day, clear and bright. Birds sounded loudly. The fields behind the diner were blanketed in a thin sheet of white frost. Elsbeth got into the car and found her father's hunting rifle and a box of bullets on the front seat—this is what he

must have gone back inside the house to get that morning.
She pushed the gun to one side and held the box of bullets
on her lap. Her father got into the car carefully. He did not
say anything about the gun. He drove along the main road
out of town, past the church. They picked up speed on the
open road, and her father smiled at her—a real smile of
release, of freedom. Anything was possible, he seemed to
say. Death can be cheated. The stories told by fathers to
daughters are true. Pumpkins can be turned into coaches,
giants overcome, miraculous escapes engineered if you are
prepared to believe. She tasted pancakes and syrup on her
tongue, looked out at the fields covered in white frost. Still-
ness. Constancy. For a few minutes in the car she felt happy.
There were places of safety and sanctuary in the everyday,
she knew that: the warm brightness of the diner, the feel of
the car seat against her legs, stalks of dry grass arcing in the
wind along the side of the road, ordinary things. Things she
could see and touch.

She felt the weight of the bullets on her lap.

"You going hunting?" she asked.

"You never know," her father said after a long time.

The fall her father died, she walked around the house at
night. Nighttime was the only time she felt calm then. As if
events had been temporarily postponed. She walked in the
dark. She listened at her father's door. She pulled on her
boots and jacket and went outside into the cold clear air.
She walked out along the white road as long as she could
stand it, and then back. One night when her father was very
sick, she saw light coming from the dining room windows.
The red velvet curtains had not closed properly and cast a
knife-edge of light across the driveway. Elsbeth looked

through the curtains and saw Lily undressing for bed. She watched her take off her uniform and underwear, then unscrew the cap of her bottle of skin cream and rub the cream in all over. She rubbed slowly, even sensuously, and looked quite different out of her clothes. Elsbeth recognized that she was beautiful. She had a different body from that of her mother—she was tall and lean and full breasted, with narrow hips and thin legs and a flat belly (horizontal scar from the hysterectomy barely visible). She was pretty, too, with her brown hair combed out. Beautiful. Lily pulled on the nightgown and the robe and knelt by the bed with her Bible. It made Elsbeth ashamed to see Lily as she was seen by those that she loved. A sister. Mortal. Flesh and blood. There were mysteries in Lily, she understood that, complexities. A person who concealed her own beauty, accepted poverty, denied herself. Here she was, tending her own dying brother, praying for him, showing a kind of restraint and courage that Elsbeth thought she would never have. She felt something expand inside her, a sadness, a yearning, something she could not define. Her father lay upstairs. The dew was falling; the hollow of the night surrounded her. The light from the window fell on the cold ground. That light would be seen for miles across the flat, hard country, from the frozen fields and from the forest on the distant hill, the light across the dark fields coming in patches through the shifting trees and falling on the still forest floor. Elsbeth turned from the window. She walked quickly down the long white road again, determined to go as fast and as far as she could before the cold became unbearable.

About the Authors

ETHAN CANIN has been the recipient of numerous literary prizes. He graduated from Stanford University with a degree in English, and then enrolled in the M.F.A. program at the Iowa Writers' Workshop. After earning an M.D. at Harvard Medical School in 1991, he began an internal medicine residency at the University of California, San Francisco. He continued to write and to practice medicine, but following the publication of his book *The Palace Thief* in 1994, he decided to concentrate on writing. In 1998, he joined the Iowa Writers' Workshop faculty. He is the author of two collections of stories, *Emperor of the Air* and *The Palace Thief*, and four novels, *Blue River, For Kings and Planets, Carry Me Across the Water,* and *America, America*. With his wife and three children, he divides his time between Iowa City and the woods of northern Michigan.

PAULINE W. CHEN attended Harvard University and the Feinberg School of Medicine, Northwestern University, and completed her surgical training at Yale University, the National Cancer Institute (National Institutes of Health), and the University of California, Los Angeles, where she was most recently a member of the faculty. In 1999, she was named the UCLA Outstanding Physician of the Year. Her first nationally published piece, "Dead Enough? The Paradox of Brain Death," appeared in the fall 2005 issue of the *Virginia Quarterly Review* and was a finalist for a 2006 National Magazine Award. She is also the 2005 cowinner of the Staige D. Blackford Prize for Nonfiction and was a finalist for the 2002 James Kirkwood Literary Prize in Creative Writing. She lives near Boston with her husband and children.

NICK EARLS graduated in medicine from the University of Queensland. He worked in general practice and as a medical editor before becoming a full-time writer of fiction in 1998. He is the author of thirteen books, including bestselling novels such as *Zigzag Street, Bachelor Kisses, Perfect Skin,* and *The True Story of Butterfish. Zigzag Street* won a Betty Trask Award in the UK in 1998, and is currently being developed into a feature film. He was the founding chair of the Australian arm of the international aid agency War Child, and is now a War Child ambassador. He has also been a patron of Kids Who Make a Difference and Hands on Art, and an honorary ambassador for the Mater Foundation, the Abused Child Trust, and the Pyjama Foundation.

ATUL GAWANDE, a surgeon and writer, is a staff member of Brigham and Women's Hospital and the Dana Farber Cancer Institute. He is also a staff writer for the *New Yorker,* Associate Professor of Surgery at Harvard Medical School, and Associate Professor in the Department of Health Policy and Management at the Harvard School of Public Health. In addition, he is the director of the World Health Organization's Global Patient Safety Challenge Safe Surgery Saves Lives. Gawande received his B.A.S. from Stanford University, M.A. (in politics, philosophy, and economics) from Oxford University, M.D. from Harvard Medical School, and M.P.H. from the Harvard School of Public Health. He served as a senior health policy advisor in the Clinton presidential campaign and in the White House from 1992 to 1993. His book *Complications: A Surgeon's Notes on an Imperfect Science* was a finalist for the National Book Award in 2002, and is published in more than a hundred countries. In 2006, he received the MacArthur Fellowship Award for his research and writing. His book *Better: A Surgeon's Notes on Performance* was a *New York Times* best seller and was one of Amazon.com's ten best books of 2007. His newest book is *The Checklist Manifesto: How to Get Things Right*. He lives in Boston with his wife and three children.

PETER GOLDSWORTHY was born in Minlaton, South Australia. He grew up in various country towns, finishing his schooling in Darwin. He graduated in medicine from the University of Adelaide in 1974, and worked for many years in alcohol and drug rehabilitation. Since then, he has divided his time evenly between writing and general practice. He has won major literary awards across a range of genres, including fiction, poetry, opera, and theater. These include the Commonwealth Poetry Prize, the FAW Christina Stead Award for Fiction, and an Australian Bicentennial Literary Award. He has published four collections of poetry, including *This Goes With That: Selected Poems 1970–1990* and *If, Then;* five collections of short fiction, including *Gravel* and *Little Deaths;* and seven novels, including *Maestro, Honk if You Are Jesus, Wish, Three Dog Night, Jesus Wants Me for a Sunbeam,* and *Everything I Knew.* He wrote the libretto for Richard Mills's opera based on Ray Lawler's play *The Summer of the Seventeenth Doll*. He has also written a comic novel, *Magpie*, jointly with Brian Matthews. He lives in Adelaide and has three children.

JEROME GROOPMAN is Professor of Medicine at Harvard Medical School, Chief of Experimental Medicine at Beth Israel Deaconess Medical Center, and one of the world's leading researchers in cancer and AIDS. He is a staff writer for the *New Yorker* and has written for the *New York Times* and the *Washington Post*. He is the author of *The Measure of Our Days, Second Opinions, An Anatomy of Hope,* and *How Doctors Think*.

JACINTA HALLORAN, a general practitioner and writer, graduated in medicine from Monash University, Melbourne. She has written on medical topics for a wide variety of publications, including the *Sunday Age* and *Inside Story*. In 2005, her short story "Finding Joshua" won the inaugural *Australian Doctor* GP Writer of the Year Award. In 2007, her novel, *Dissection,* was shortlisted for the Victorian Premier's Literary Prize for an Unpublished Manuscript; in 2008, it was published by Scribe Publications. She completed an M.A. in creative writing at RMIT University in 2009. She is currently writing her second novel, and lives in Melbourne with her husband and three children.

SANDEEP JAUHAR is a cardiologist and the director of the Heart Failure Program at Long Island Jewish Medical Center. Before graduating from medical school at Washington University in St. Louis, he received a Ph.D. in condensed matter physics from the University of California, Berkeley. He writes regularly for the *New York Times* and the *New England Journal of Medicine*. He is the recipient of a SAJA

Journalism Award for outstanding stories about medicine. His first book, *Intern: A Doctor's Initiation,* was a US best seller, and has been published in many countries. He lives with his wife and their two children in Old Brookville, New York.

PERRI KLASS is Professor of Journalism and Pediatrics at New York University. She attended Harvard Medical School and completed her residency in pediatrics at Children's Hospital, Boston, and her fellowship in pediatric infectious diseases at Boston City Hospital. She has written extensively about medicine, children, literacy, and knitting. Her nonfiction includes *Every Mother Is a Daughter: The Neverending Quest for Success, Inner Peace, and a Really Clean Kitchen,* which she coauthored with her mother, Sheila Solomon Klass, and *Quirky Kids: Understanding and Helping Your Child Who Doesn't Fit In,* which she coauthored with Eileen Costello. She is also the author of two collections and other works of fiction including the novels *The Mystery of Breathing* and *Other Women's Children.* Her most recent books are *Treatment Kind and Fair: Letters to a Young Doctor* and *The Mercy Rule.* Her short stories have won five O. Henry awards, and in 2006 she was the recipient of the Women's National Book Association Award. She is a longtime member of the executive board of PEN New England, which she chaired from 2004 to 2006.

ROBERT JAY LIFTON was born in New York City and graduated from New York Medical College in 1948. He completed his training in psychiatry at the Downstate Medical Center, Brooklyn, New York. He was an air force psychiatrist serving in the United States, Japan, and Korea from 1951 to 1953. He was research associate in psychiatry at

Harvard from 1956 to 1961. He is a visiting professor of psychiatry at Harvard Medical School and Cambridge Hospital, a former distinguished professor of psychiatry and psychology at the Graduate School University Center, and director of the Center on Violence and Human Survival at John Jay College of Criminal Justice at the City University of New York. He is the author of many books including *The Nazi Doctors: Medical Killing and the Psychology of Genocide; Death in Life: Survivors and Hiroshima; Destroying the World to Save It: Aum Shinrikyo, Apocalyptic Violence, and the New Global Terrorism; Hiroshima in America: Fifty Years of Denial* (with Greg Mitchell); and *The Protean Self: Human Resilience in an Age of Fragmentation.*

JOHN MURRAY was born in Adelaide, South Australia, where he studied medicine. He has an M.P.H. from Johns Hopkins University and is a graduate of the Iowa Writers' Workshop, where he was a teaching-writing fellow. In 1992, he joined the Epidemic Intelligence Service of the Centers for Disease Control and Prevention, specializing in epidemic dysentery and cholera in Africa and Asia. Since 1995, he has worked full-time on child health programs in developing countries, most recently in China and Ghana. He is the author of *A Few Short Notes on Tropical Butterflies.*

DANIELLE OFRI is Associate Professor of Medicine at New York University School of Medicine, but her clinical home is at Bellevue Hospital, the oldest public hospital in the United States. She is cofounder and editor in chief of the *Bellevue Literary Review.* Her newest book, *Medicine in Translation: Journeys with My Patients,* is about the experience of immigrants and Americans in the US health care system. She is the author of two collections of essays about life in medicine: *Incidental Findings: Lessons from My Patients in the Art of Medicine* and *Singular Intimacies: Becoming a Doctor at Bellevue.* She also edited *The Best of the Bellevue Literary Review.* Her writings have appeared in the *New York Times,* the *Los Angeles Times,* the *New England Journal of Medicine,* and the *Lancet,* and on National Public Radio. Her essays have been selected for *Best American Essays* (twice) and *Best American Science Writing.* She is the recipient of the John P. McGovern Award from the American Medical Writers Association for "pre-eminent contributions to medical communication."

OLIVER SACKS was born in London, to a family of physicians and scientists. He studied at Oxford University and did residencies and fellowship work at Mt. Zion Hospital in San Francisco and at the University of California, Los Angeles. He has lived and worked in New York since 1965. In 2007, he was appointed Professor of Neurology and Psychiatry at Columbia University Medical Center, and was also designated the university's first Columbia University Artist. In 1966, he began working as a consulting neurologist for Beth Abraham Hospital in the Bronx, a chronic care hospital; there he encountered an extraordinary group of patients, later to become the subjects of his well-known book *Awakenings,* which inspired a play by Harold Pinter (*A Kind of Alaska*) and the Oscar-nominated feature film *Awakenings,* starring Robert De Niro and Robin Williams. Sacks is also known for his collections *The Man Who Mistook His Wife for a Hat* and *An Anthropologist on Mars,* in which he describes patients struggling to live with a range of often bizarre neurological conditions. He has written about the world of the deaf and sign language in *Seeing Voices,* and about a community of color-blind people in *The Island of the Colorblind.* He has explored his experiences as a doctor in *Migraine,* and as a patient in *A Leg to Stand On.* His autobiography, *Uncle Tungsten: Memories of a Chemical Boyhood,* was published in 2001. His most recent book is *Musicophilia: Tales of Music and the Brain.* His work, which has been supported by the Guggenheim Foundation and the Alfred P. Sloan Foundation, regularly appears in the *New Yorker* and the *New York Review of Books,* as well as in medical journals. The *New York Times* has referred to him as "the poet laureate of medicine," and in 2002, he was awarded Rockefeller University's Lewis Thomas Prize, which recognizes the scientist as poet. He is an honorary fellow of both the American Academy of Arts and Letters and the American Academy of Arts and Sciences, and holds honorary degrees from many universities and colleges, including Oxford, the Karolinska Institute, Georgetown, Bard, Gallaudet, Tufts, and the Catholic University of Peru.

ABRAHAM VERGHESE is Professor for the Theory and Practice of Medicine at the Stanford University School of Medicine, and Senior Associate Chair of the Department of Internal Medicine. Born of Indian parents, he grew up near Addis Ababa, Ethiopia, and began his medical training there. After moving to the US, he took time off from medicine to study writing at the Iowa Writers' Workshop at the University of Iowa, where he earned an M.F.A. in 1991. Since then, his writing has appeared in the *New Yorker, Texas Monthly, Granta,* the *Atlantic, Forbes.com,* the *New York Times,* the *New York Times Magazine,* and the *Wall Street Journal,* among others. His first book, *My Own Country: A Doctor's Story of a Town and Its People in the Age of Aids,* published in 1994, was one of five chosen as best books of the year by *Time* magazine, and later was made into a TV movie directed by Mira Nair. His second book, *The Tennis Partner: A Story of Friendship and Loss,* about his friend and tennis partner's struggle with addiction, was a *New York Times* Notable Book. *Cutting for Stone,* his first novel, was published in 2009, and was a *New York Times* best seller.

GABRIEL WESTON was born in London. She earned an M.A. in English literature at Edinburgh University and studied medicine in London. She qualified as a doctor in 2000, and became a Member of the Royal College of Surgeons in 2003. Her collection *Direct Red: A Surgeon's Story* was longlisted for the Guardian First Book Award. She works as a part-time ENT surgeon and is writing her second book. She lives in London with her husband and two children.

IRVIN YALOM was born in Washington, DC, and graduated from Boston University School of Medicine. He is Emeritus Professor of Psychiatry at Stanford University School of Medicine, and is the author of the classic textbooks *The Theory and Practice of Group Psychotherapy, Existential Psychotherapy,* and *Inpatient Group Psychotherapy,* and coauthor of *Every Day Gets a Little Closer, Encounter Groups: First Facts,* and *A Concise Guide to Group Psychotherapy.* He has also written *Love's Executioner, Momma and the Meaning of Life* (a collection of true and fictionalized tales of therapy), *Staring at the Sun: Overcoming the Terror of Death,* and three novels, *When Nietzsche Wept, Lying on the Couch,* and *The Schopenhauer Cure. The Yalom Reader* is an anthology of his best-known works, and he has also written a collection of essays on writing. He is married and has four children.

Acknowledgments

This project would not have been possible without the help and support of many people. First and foremost, I am indebted to the incredible generosity of all the contributors to this anthology. I would also like to thank Peter Balakian, Peter Bishop, Lexy Bloom, Lan Samantha Chang, Evan Fallenberg, Deborah Harris, Robin Hemley, Carolyn Hessel, Antoni Jach, Edward Kastenmeier, Lee Kofman, Michael Kramer, Judy Labensohn, Bev Magennis, Nicola Redhouse, Henry Rosenbloom, Todd Shuster, Amanda Tokar, and Danny Yanez. Special thanks to Jacinta Dimase, Donna-Lee Frieze, Diana Hanaor, Deborah Leiser-Moore, and Sandra Levin.

"Falling Down" from *Intern: A Doctor's Initiation* by Sandeep Jauhar, copyright © 2008 by Sandeep Jauhar. Reprinted by permission of Farrar, Straus and Giroux, LLC, New York.

"Tahirih" by Leah Kaminsky, copyright © 2009 by Leah Kaminsky. First published in *Transnational Literature 2*, Flinders University, Adelaide.

"Index Case" by Perri Klass, copyright © 2004 by Massachusetts Medical Society. All rights reserved. First published in *The New England Journal of Medicine* Vol. 350, 5/13/2004. Reprinted by permission of Massachusetts Medical Society.

"The Infernal Chorus" from *Witness to an Extreme Century: A Memoir* by Robert Jay Lifton, copyright © 2011 by Robert Jay Lifton. Reprinted by permission of Free Press, a division of Simon & Schuster, Inc., New York.

"Communion" by John Murray, copyright © 2010 by John Murray. Reprinted by permission of John Murray.

"Intensive Care" from *Singular Intimacies: Becoming a Doctor at Bellevue* by Danielle Ofri, copyright © 2003 by Danielle Ofri. Reprinted by permission of Beacon Press, Boston.

"The Lost Mariner" from *The Man Who Mistook His Wife for a Hat and Other Clinical Tales* by Oliver Sacks, copyright © 1970, 1981, 1983, 1984, 1985 by Oliver Sacks. Reprinted by permission of Simon & Schuster, Inc., New York, and Pan MacMillan, London.

"Bedside Manners" by Abraham Verghese, copyright © 2007 by Abraham Verghese. First published in *Texas Monthly*, 2007. Reprinted by permission of *Texas Monthly* and Abraham Verghese.

"Beauty" from *Direct Red* by Gabriel Weston, copyright © 2009 by Gabriel Weston. Reprinted by permission of HarperCollins Publishers, New York; Jonathan Cape, a division of The Random House Group Ltd., London; and Doubleday Canada, Toronto.

"Do Not Go Gentle" from *Love's Executioner and Other Tales of Psychotherapy* by Irvin D. Yalom, copyright © 1989 by Irvin D. Yalom. Reprinted by permission of Basic Books, a member of the Perseus Books Group, New York, and Penguin Books Ltd., London.